SHANKARA'S

# CREST-JEWEL
# OF DISCRIMINATION

The following titles by Swami Prabhavananda are
   suggested for further reading:

*Original Works*

Vedic Religion and Philosophy
The Eternal Companion
The Spiritual Heritage of India (with Frederick
   Manchester)
Sermon on the Mount According to Vedanta
Religion in  Practice
Yoga and Mysticism

*Translations*

Bhagavad Gita: The Song of God (with
   Christopher Isherwood)
The Upanishads: Breath of the Eternal (with
   Frederick Manchester)
Srimad Bhagavatam: The Wisdom of God
How to Know God: The Yoga Aphorisms of
   Patanjali (with Christopher Isherwood)

*by Christopher Isherwood*
Ramakrishna and His Disciples

SHANKARA'S

# Crest-Jewel
# of Discrimination

*(Viveka-Chudamani)*

Translated
with an Introduction to
Shankara's Philosophy

## by Swami Prabhavananda

## and Christopher Isherwood

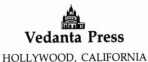

**Vedanta Press**

HOLLYWOOD, CALIFORNIA

ISBN: 0-87481-034-5
Library of Congress Catalog Card Number 78-51354
Vedanta Press, Hollywood, California 90068

First Edition published 1947. Third Edition 1978
Printed in the United States of America

Readers interested in the subject matter of this
book are invited to correspond with The Secre-
tary, Vedanta Society of Southern California, 1946
Vedanta Place, Hollywood, CA 90068.

# Contents

Oh Lord, dweller within;
You are the light
In the heart's lotus.
Om is your very self,
Om, holiest word,
Seed and source of the scriptures.
Logic cannot discover
You, Lord, but the yogis
Know you in meditation.
In you are all God's faces,
His forms and aspects,
In you also
We find the guru.
In every heart you are
And if but once, only,
A man will open
His mind to receive you
Truly that man
Is free forever.

—*Shankara.*

# I

# Shankara

BEAUTIFUL and fantastic clouds of legend sur-
round the austere, charming, boyish figure of
Shankara—saint, philosopher and poet. But, his-
torically speaking, we know very little about the
circumstances of his life.

He was born in or around the year 686 A.D. of
Brahmin parents, at Kaladi, a small village of
Western Malabar, in southern India. By the age of
ten, he was already an academic prodigy. Not
only had he read and memorized all the scriptures, but he had written commentaries on many
of them, and had held discussions with famous
scholars who came to him from every part of the
country.

Yet the boy was dissatisfied. At a time when
most children are only beginning to study, he was
already disgusted by the emptiness of book-
knowledge. He saw that his teachers did not
practice the lofty truths they preached. Indeed,
the whole society in which he lived was
materialistic and pleasure-seeking. India was
passing through a period of spiritual decadence.
Shankara, burning with youthful zeal, resolved to

make his own life an example which would lead men back to the paths of truth.

At this period, his father died. The boy puzzled over the riddle of life and death, and determined to solve it. He would renounce everything in his search for the meaning of existence. It was then he wrote the poem called *Moha Mudgaram*—"The Shattering of Illusion." Here is a more or less literal translation:

Who is thy wife? Who is thy son?
The ways of this world are strange indeed.
Whose art thou? Whence art thou come?
Vast is thy ignorance, my beloved.
Therefore ponder these things and worship the
    Lord.

Behold the folly of Man:
In childhood busy with his toys,
In youth bewitched by love,
In age bowed down with cares—
And always unmindful of the Lord!
The hours fly, the seasons roll, life ebbs,
But the breeze of hope blows continually in his
    heart.

Birth brings death, death brings rebirth:
This evil needs no proof.
Where then O Man, is thy happiness?
This life trembles in the balance
Like water on a lotus-leaf—
And yet the sage can show us, in an instant,
How to bridge this sea of change.

When the body is wrinkled, when the hair
  turns grey,
When the gums are toothless, and the old
  man's staff
Shakes like a reed beneath his weight,
The cup of his desire is still full.

Thy son may bring thee suffering,
Thy wealth is no assurance of heaven:
Therefore be not vain of thy wealth,
Or of thy family, or of thy youth—
All are fleeting, all must change.
Know this and be free.
Enter the joy of the Lord.

Seek neither peace nor strife
With kith or kin, with friend or foe.
O beloved, if thou wouldst attain freedom,
Be equal unto all.

Shankara now persuaded his mother to let him take the monastic vow, promising that he would return to visit her before she died. Then, having made arrangements for her needs, he set out in search of a teacher.

On the banks of the river Narmada, he met Gaudapada, a famous philosopher and seer, who had attained knowledge of the Reality. Shankara asked the old man for initiation, but Gaudapada refused. He had made a vow to remain absorbed in union with Brahman. However, he sent the boy to his foremost disciple, Govindapada. Govindapada initiated him and instructed him in meditation and the whole process of Yoga. Within a very short time, Shankara achieved complete mystical realization, and himself went out to teach.

One morning, when he was on his way to bathe in the Ganges, he met a *Chandala*, a member of the lowest caste, the untouchables. The man had four dogs with him, and they were blocking Shankara's path. For a moment, inborn caste-prejudice asserted itself. Shankara, the Brahmin, ordered the *Chandala* out of his way. But the *Chandala* answered: "If there is only one God, how can there be many kinds of men?" Shankara was filled with shame and reverence. He prostrated himself before the *Chandala*. This incident inspired one of Shankara's finest poems, the *Manisha Panchaka*—It consists of five stanzas, each one ending with the refrain:

> He who has learned to see the one Existence everywhere,
> He is my master—be he Brahmin or Chandala.

Shankara began his teaching among the scholars of the country, converting the teachers first, and then their pupils. One of them was the famous philospher Mandan Misra. Mandan Misra held that the life of the householder was far superior to that of the monk, and his opinion was respected and widely shared throughout India. Shankara determined to argue with him, and journeyed to his home. When he arrived, he found the doors locked. Misra was holding a religious ceremony and did not wish to be disturbed. Shankara, with the mischievous spirit of a boy in his teens, climbed a nearby tree and jumped down from it into the courtyard. Misra noticed him among the crowd. He disapproved of monks—especially when they were so youthful—and asked sarcastically: "Whence comes this shaven head?" "You have eyes to see, Sir," Shankara answered saucily: "The shaven head comes up from the neck." Misra lost his temper, but Shankara continued to tease him, and at length the two of them agreed to hold a debate on the relative merits of the monk's and householder's lives. It was understood that Shankara, if he lost, should become a householder, and that Misra, if he lost, should become a monk. The debate lasted for several days. Bharati, the learned wife of Misra, acted as umpire. Finally, Shankara was able to convince Misra of the superiority of the monastic life, and Misra became his disciple. It was he who later annotated Shankara's commentaries on the Brahma-Sutras.

Shankara's life came to an end at Kedarnath in the Himalayas. He was only thirty-two years old. During this brief period, he had established many monasteries, and had founded ten monastic orders. This was the first time that monasticism had ever been organized in India, and Shankara's system still exists at the present day. He was a reformer rather than an innovator. He preached no new doctrine or creed. But he gave a new impulse to the spiritual life of his time. Separated by intervals of a thousand years, like three tremendous mountain peaks, Buddha, Shankara and Ramakrishna dominate the range of India's religious history.

Shankara's literary output was enormous. He not only made commentaries on the Vedanta Sutras, the principal Upanishads and the Bhagavad-Gita, but produced two major philosophical works, the Upadeshasahasri and the Vivekachudamani (the Crest-Jewel of Discrimination.) He was also the author of many poems, hymns, prayers, and minor works on Vedanta.

The Crest-Jewel of Discrimination is written entirely in verse; possibly because this would be easier for pupils to memorize. The lines are long and the metre is intricate; we have decided not to attempt to reproduce it in English. Shankara's message is infinitely more important than its literary form: clarity has been our only aim throughout the text. For this reason, we have not hesitated to paraphrase and expand whenever necessary; but the translation remains, on the whole, very close to the original.

# II

SHANKARA'S

# Philosophy of Non-Dualism

## The Spirit of Shankara's Philosophy

"BRAHMAN—the absolute existence, knowledge and bliss—is real. The universe is not real. Brahman and Atman (man's inner Self) are one."

In these words, Shankara sums up his philosophy. What are the implications of this statement? What does he mean by "real" and by "not real"?

Shankara only accepts as "real" that which neither changes nor ceases to exist. In making this definition, he follows the teachings of the Upanishads and of Gaudapada, his predecessor. No object, no kind of knowledge, can be absolutely real if its existence is only temporary. Absolute reality implies permanent existence. If we consider our various experiences during the states of waking and dreaming, we find that dream-experiences are contradicted by waking-experiences and vice versa—and that both kinds of experience cease in dreamless sleep. In other words, every object of knowledge, external or internal—for a thought or idea is as much an object of knowledge as is the external world—is subject to modification and therefore, by Shankara's definition, "not real".

What, then, *is* the Reality behind all our experiences? There is only one thing that never leaves us—the deep consciousness. This alone is the constant feature of all experience. And this consciousness is the real, absolute Self. In dreamless sleep, also, the real Self is present as a witness, while the ego-sense which we call "ourself", our individuality, has become temporarily merged in ignorance (avidya) and disappeared.

Vedanta Philosophy occupies a central position between realism and idealism. Western realism and idealism are both based on a distinction between mind and matter; Indian philosophy puts mind and matter in the same category—both are objects of knowledge. Shankara should not, however, be regarded as a precursor of Berkeley: he does not say that the world is unreal simply because its existence depends upon our perception. The world, according to Shankara, "is and is not". Its fundamental unreality can only be understood in reference to the ultimate mystical experience, the experience of an illumined soul. When the illumined soul passes into transcendental consciousness, he realizes the Self (the Atman) as pure bliss and pure intelligence, the "One without a second". In this state of consciousness, all perception of multiplicity ceases, there is no longer any sense of "mine" and "thine", the world as we ordinarily know it has vanished.

Then the Self shines forth as the One, the Truth, the Brahman, the basis of this world-appearance. World-appearance as it is experienced in the waking state may be likened, says Shankara, to an imagined snake which proves, on closer inspection, to be nothing but a coil of rope. When the truth is known, we are no longer deluded by the appearance—the snake-appearance vanishes into the reality of the rope, the world vanishes into Brahman.

Other systems of Hindu philosophy—Sankhya, Yoga or Nyaya—maintain that the phenomenal world possesses an objective reality, even though it may not be apparent to the eyes of an illumined soul. Advaita Vedanta differs from them on this vital point: it denies the ultimate reality of the world of thought and matter. Mind and matter, finite objects and their relations, are a misreading of Brahman, and nothing more—that is what Shankara teaches.

## The Nature of World-Appearance

When Shankara says that the world of thought and matter is not real, he does not mean that it is non-existent. The world-appearance is and is not. In the state of ignorance (our everyday consciousness) it is experienced, and it exists as it appears. In the state of illumination it is not experienced, and it ceases to exist. Shankara does not regard any experience as non-existent as long as it is experienced, but he very naturally draws a distinction between the private illusions of the individual and the universal or world-illusion. The former he calls pratibhasika (illusory) and the latter vyavaharika (phenomenal). For example, a man's dreams are his private illusions; when he wakes, they cease. But the universal illusion—the illusion of world-phenomena—continues throughout a man's whole waking life; unless he becomes aware of the Truth through knowledge of Brahman. Shankara makes, also, a further distinction between these two kinds of illusion and those ideas which are altogether unreal and imaginary, which represent a total impossibility or a flat contradiction in terms—such as the son of a barren woman.

Here, then, we are confronted by a paradox— the world is and is not. It is neither real nor non-existent. And yet this apparent paradox is simply a statement of fact—a fact which Shankara calls Maya. This Maya, this world-appearance, has its basis in Brahman, the eternal. The concept of Maya applies only to the phenomenal world, which, according to Shankara, consists of names and forms. It is not non-existent, yet it differs from the Reality, the Brahman, upon which it depends for its existence. It is not real, since it disappears in the light of knowledge of its eternal basis. World-appearance is Maya; the Self, the Atman, alone is real.

## Superimposition, or Maya

The most difficult of all philosophical problems is the relation between the finite and the Infinite; the problem of how this finite world came into being. If we believe that the finite has an absolute reality of its own and that it has emerged from the Infinite and is an actual transformation of the Infinite, or if we regard the Infinite as a transcendental first cause of the phenomenal world (a position held by most Christian theologians), then we must admit that the Infinite is infinite no longer. A God who transforms Himself into the visible universe is Himself subject to transformation and change—He cannot be regarded as the absolute reality. A God who creates a world limits Himself by the very act of creation, and thus ceases to be infinite. The question, "Why should God create at all?" remains unanswered.

This difficulty is overcome, however, if we consider the world as Maya. And this explanation of our universe is, moreover, in perfect accord with the findings of modern science—which may be summarized as follows:

"A soap-bubble with irregularities and corrugations on its surface is perhaps the best representation of the new universe revealed to us by the theory of relativity. The universe is not the interior of the soap-bubble but its surface—and the substance out of which this bubble is blown, the soap film, is empty space welded into empty time."[1]

Thus it is only when we analyze the nature of the universe and discover it to be Maya—neither absolutely real nor absolutely non-existent—that we learn how the phenomenal surface of the soap-bubble safeguards the eternal presence of the Absolute.

[1]Sir James Jeans.

The Upanishads, it is true, appear to consider Brahman as the first cause of the universe, both material and efficient. They declare that the universe emanates from, subsists in and finally merges into the absolute Brahman. Shankara never directly contradicts the Upanishads, but he explains such statements in a different way. The universe, he says, is a superimposition upon Brahman. Brahman remains eternally infinite and unchanged. It is not transformed into this universe. It simply *appears* as this universe to us, in our ignorance. We superimpose the apparent world upon Brahman, just as we sometimes superimpose a snake upon a coil of rope.

This theory of superimposition (vivartavada) is inseparably linked with the theory of causality. Causal relation exists in the world of multiplicity, which is Maya. Within Maya, the mind cannot function without causal relation. But to speak of cause and effect with reference to the Absolute is simply absurd. To seek to know what caused the world is to transcend the world, to seek to find the cause of Maya is to go beyond Maya—and, when we do that, Maya vanishes, for the effect ceases to exist. How, then, can there be a cause of a non-existent effect? In other words, the relation between Brahman and Maya is, by its very nature, unknowable and indefinable by any process of the human intellect.

## Maya: A Statement of Fact as Well as a Principle

Thus, according to Shankara, the world of thought and matter has a phenomenal or relative existence, and is superimposed upon Brahman, the unique, absolute reality. As long as we remain in ignorance (i.e., as long as we have not achieved transcendental consciousness) we shall continue to experience this apparent world which is the effect of superimposition. When transcendental consciousness is achieved, superimposition ceases.

What is the nature of this superimposition? In the introduction to his commentary on the Brahma Sutras, Shankara tells us that "Superimposition is the apparent presentation to consciousness, by the memory, of something previously observed elsewhere." We see a snake. We remember it. Next day, we see a coil of rope. We superimpose the remembered snake upon it, and thereby misunderstand its nature.

Shankara foresees an objection to his theory and goes on to anticipate and answer it. We may challenge the theory of superimposition by pointing out that Brahman is not an object of perception. How can we superimpose a snake upon a rope which we do not perceive? How can we superimpose a world-appearance upon a reality which is not apparent to our senses? "For every man superimposes objects only upon such other objects as are placed before him (i.e., as come into contact with his sense-organs)." To this, Shankara answers: "Brahman is not, we reply, non-objective in the absolute sense. For Brahman is the object of the ego-idea. We know quite well, by intuition, that the inner Self must exist, since the ego-idea is a presentation of the Self. Nor is it an absolute rule that objects can be superimposed only upon such other objects as are placed before us; for ignorant people superimpose a dark-blue color upon the sky, which is not an object of sense-perception."

This statement needs some further explanation. Although Brahman is never apparent to our everyday sense-perception, there *is* a manner in which we are aware of the reality, the inner Self. Brahman, it has been said, is absolute existence, knowledge and bliss. Only in transcendental consciousness can we know this fully. Yet Brahman is partly apparent to our normal consciousness also. Brahman is Existence, and we all know that we exist. In this sense, every one of us has an intuitive knowledge of the inner Self (the Atman, or Brahman-within-the-creature). The inner Self, the reality, is never an object of sense-perception, however,—because, in our ignorance, we superimpose the idea of a private individuality— of being Mr. Smith or Mrs. Jones—upon our awareness of Existence. We are unable to understand that Existence is not our private property, that it is universal and absolute. The inner Self is therefore present in our normal consciousness as "the object of the ego-idea"—a literal translation of Shankara's phrase. The superimposition of the ego-idea upon Existence is our first and most important act as human beings. The moment we have made this central act of superimposition— the moment we have said, "I am I, I am private, I am separate, I am an individual"—we have set up a kind of chain-reaction which makes further superimposition inevitable. The claim to individuality for ourselves implies individuality everywhere. It automatically superimposes a multiple world of creatures and objects upon the one, undivided reality, the Existence which is Brahman. Ego-idea and world-appearance depend upon each other. Lose the ego-idea in transcendental consciousness, and the world-appearance must necessarily vanish.

When and how did this act of superimposition occur? Was it at our individual birth, or in some previous life? Was there an historical moment—corresponding to the story of the fall of Adam—at which the phenomenal world came into being as the result of the ego-idea? The futility of such questions should be self-evident. We merely go round in a circle. What is this world-appearance? Maya. What causes it? Our ignorance. What is this ignorance? Maya, also. If there was, and is and always will be one unchanging reality, how can we possibly assume that Maya began at some definite historical moment in time? We cannot.

Therefore, we are forced to conclude, as Shankara does, that Maya, like Brahman, is without any beginning. Ignorance as the cause and world-appearance as the effect have existed always and will always exist. They are like seed and tree. The "coupling of the real and the unreal", produced by our ignorance, is a process universally evident in our daily lives. Shankara says: "It is obvious and needs no proof that the object which is the non-ego and the subject which is the ego-idea (superimposed upon the Self) are opposed to each other, like light and darkness, and cannot be identified. Still less can their respective attributes be identified. . . . Nevertheless, it is natural to man (because of his wrong knowledge) not to be able to distinguish between these distinct entities and their respective attributes. He superimposes upon each the nature and attributes of the other, coupling the real with the unreal, and making use of such expressions as 'I am that', 'that is mine'."

Shankara is speaking here of two stages in the process of superimposition. First, the ego idea is superimposed upon the inner Self, the existence-reality. Then the ego-idea, reaching outward, as it were, identifies itself with the body and the body's mental and physical attributes and actions. We say, as a matter of course, "I am fat", "I am tired", "I am walking", "I am sitting down"— without ever stopping to consider what this "I" really is. We go further. We claim purely external objects and conditions for our own. We announce that "I am a Republican", or that "this house is mine". As superimpositions multiply, extra-ordinary statements become possible and nor-mal—such as "we sunk three submarines yester-day" or "I carry a good deal of insurance". We identify our ego, more or less, with every object in the universe. And all the while, the inner Self looks on, utterly detached from these moods and antics—yet making them all possible, by lending to the mind that light of consciousness without which Maya could not exist.

That Maya is beginningless can also be shown if we return for a moment to the image of the rope and the snake. The superimposition of the snake upon the rope is only possible if we can re-member what a snake looks like; a child who had never seen a snake could never superimpose it. How then is it possible for the newly-born child to superimpose the "snake" (world-appearance) upon the "rope" (Brahman)? We can only answer this question if we postulate a universal "snake-memory", which is common to all mankind, and has existed from a time without beginning. This "snake-memory" is Maya.

Maya, says Shankara, is not only universal but beginningless and endless. A distinction must, however, be made between Maya as a universal principle and ignorance (avidya) which is individual. Individual ignorance is beginningless, but it can end at any moment: it is lost when a man achieves spiritual illumination. Thus the world may vanish from the consciousness of an individual and yet continue to exist for the rest of mankind. In saying this, Shankara's philosophy differs essentially from the subjective idealism of the West.

## Brahman and Iswara

In a sense, Brahman is the ultimate cause of the universe—since, by the action of Maya, the world-appearance is superimposed upon Brahman. Brahman is the cause, Maya the effect. Yet Brahman cannot be said to have transformed itself into the world, or to have created it, since absolute Reality is, by definition, incapable of temporal action or change. Another word, Iswara, must therefore be employed to describe the creative principle. Iswara is Brahman united with Maya—the combination of Brahman and its power which creates, preserves and dissolves the universe in an endless and beginningless process. Iswara is God personified, God with attributes.

According to the Sankhya system of philosophy, the universe is an evolution of Prakriti—undifferentiated matter, composed of three forces, called the gunas. Creation is a disturbance in the balance of these forces. The gunas begin to enter into an enormous variety of combinations—somewhat as in the western theory of atomic structure—and these combinations are individual elements, objects and creatures. This concept of Prakriti corresponds, more or less, to Shankara's concept of Maya—but with this important difference: Prakriti is said to be other than, and independent of Purusha (the absolute Reality) while Maya is said to have no absolute reality but to be dependent on Brahman. Therefore it is Iswara, rather than Prakriti, who can be described as the ultimate cause of the universe.

Are there then two Gods—one the impersonal Brahman, the other the personal Iswara? No—for Brahman only appears as Iswara when viewed by the relative ignorance of Maya. Iswara has the same degree of reality as Maya has. God the Person is not the ultimate nature of Brahman. In the words of Swami Vivekananda, "Personal God is the reading of the Impersonal by the human mind."

Sri Ramakrishna, who lived continually in the consciousness of absolute Brahman, used the following illustration: "Brahman may be compared to an infinite ocean, without beginning or end. Just as, through intense cold, some portions of the ocean freeze into ice and the formless water appears to have form, so, through the intense love of the devotee, Brahman appears to take on form and personality. But the form melts away again as the sun of knowledge rises. Then the universe also disappears, and there is seen to be nothing but Brahman, the infinite."

Although Iswara is, in a sense, a person, we must beware of regarding Him as similar to, or identical with the jiva, the individual human soul. Iswara, like the jiva, is Brahman united with Maya, but with this fundamental difference—Iswara is the ruler and controller of Maya, the jiva is Maya's servant and plaything. We can therefore say, without paradox, that we are, at the same time, God and the servants of God. In our absolute nature, we are one with Brahman; in our relative nature, we are other than the Iswara, and subject to Him.

Devotion to the Iswara, the Personal God, may lead a man very far along the path of spirituality, it may make him into a saint. But this is not the ultimate knowledge. To be completely enlightened is to go beyond Iswara, to know the Impersonal Reality behind the personal divine Appearance. We can become Brahman, since Brahman is present in us always. But we can never become Iswara, because Iswara is above and distinct from our human personality. It follows, therefore, that we can never become rulers of the universe—for that is Iswara's function. The desire to usurp the function of Iswara is the ultimate madness of ego. It is symbolized in Christian literature by the legend of the fall of Lucifer.

Vyasa, the author of the Brahma Sutras, makes

the same point when he says that no one will acquire the power of creating, ruling or dissolving the universe, since that power belongs to Iswara alone. And Shankara in his commentary discusses the problem as follows: "If a man, by worshipping the qualified Brahman (Iswara), achieves knowledge of the Supreme Ruler while still preserving his individual consciousness—is his power limited or unlimited? When this question arises, some will argue that his power is unlimited, and they will quote the scriptural texts (referring to those who achieve knowledge of Iswara) 'They attain their own kingdom', 'To them all the gods offer worship', 'Their desires are fulfilled in all the worlds.' But Vyasa answers this question when he adds, 'without the power of ruling the universe'. All the other powers of Iswara can be acquired by the liberated, but that power belongs to Iswara alone. How do we know this? Because He is the subject of the scriptural texts concerning creation. These texts do not refer to the liberated souls, in any connection whatsoever. That is why He is called 'the ever-perfect'. The scriptures also say that the powers of the liberated are acquired by worshipping and searching after God; therefore they have no place in the ruling of the universe. Again, because these liberated souls still preserve their individual consciousness, it is possible that their wills may differ, and that, while one desires creation, another may desire destruction. The only way to avoid this conflict is to make all wills subordinate to some one will. Therefore we must conclude that the wills of the liberated are dependent on the will of the Supreme Ruler."

If there is only one consciousness, one Brahman, who is the seer and who is the seen? Who sees Brahman as Iswara, and who is the jiva? Are they different or one?

As long as man is within the limitations of Maya, the One is seen as many. Ignorance can do no better than to worship Appearance; and Iswara is the ruler of all appearances—the highest idea which the human mind can grasp and the human heart can love. The human mind can never grasp the absolute Reality, it can only infer its presence and worship its projected image. In the process of this worship, the mind becomes purified, the ego-idea thins away like mist, superimposition ceases, Iswara and world-appearance both vanish in the blaze of transcendental consciousness when there is no seer, no seen—nothing but Brahman, the single, all-embracing, timeless Fact.

## The Problem of Evil

Every religion or system of philosophy has to deal with the problem of evil—and unfortunately it is a problem which is usually explained away rather than explained. "Why," it is asked, "does God permit evil, when He Himself is all goodness?"

One of two answers is usually given to this question by Western religious thought. Sometimes we are told that evil is educational and penal. God punishes us for our sins by visiting us with war, famine, earthquake, disaster and disease. He employs temptation (either directly or through the agency of the Devil) to test and strengthen the virtue of the good. This is the answer given by the Old Testament. It repels many people today and has become unfashionable—although, as we shall see in a moment, it contains a certain degree of truth, according to the philosophy of Vedanta.

The other answer—now more generally accepted—is that evil does not exist at all. If we view Life *sub specie aeternitatis*, we shall know that evil has no reality; that it is simply a misreading of good.

Vedanta Philosophy disagrees with both these answers—with the second even more radically than with the first. How it asks, can evil be changed into good, merely by viewing it in a special manner? Pain and misfortune may be borne more easily if we fix our minds upon God—but they are very real experiences nevertheless, even though their duration is limited. Vedanta agrees that evil, in the absolute sense, is unreal. But it reminds us that, from this standpoint, good is unreal also. The absolute Reality is beyond good and evil, pleasure and pain, success and disaster. Both good and evil are aspects of Maya. As long as Maya exists, they exist. Within Maya they are real enough.

The question "Why does God permit evil?" is, in fact, most misleadingly phrased. It is as absurd as if one were to ask "Why does God permit good?" Nobody today would ask why rain "permitted" a catastrophic flood; nobody would blame or praise fire because it burns one man's house and cooks another man's dinner. Nor can it be properly said that Brahman is "good" in any personal sense of the word. Brahman is not "good" in the sense that Christ was "good"—for Christ's goodness was within Maya; his life expressed the light of Reality reflected upon the relative world. The Reality itself is beyond all phenomena; even the noblest. It is beyond purity, beauty, happiness, glory or success. It can be described as "good" only if we mean that absolute consciousness is absolute knowledge, and that absolute knowledge is absolute joy.

But perhaps the question does not refer to Brahman at all. Perhaps, in this connection, "God" means Iswara, the Ruler of Maya. If this is granted, can Vedanta Philosophy agree with the Old Testament that God is a law-giver, a stern and somewhat unpredictable father, whose ways are not ours, whose punishments and rewards often seem unmerited, who permits us to fall into temptation? The answer is yes and no. The Vedanta doctrine of Karma is a doctrine of absolute, automatic justice. The circumstances of our lives, our pains and our pleasures, are all the result of our past actions in this and countless previous existences, from a beginningless time. Viewed from a relative standpoint, Maya is quite pitiless. We get exactly what we earn, no more, no less. If we cry out against some apparent injustice, it is only because the act that brought it upon us is buried deep in the past, out of reach of our memory. To be born a beggar, a king, an athlete or a helpless cripple is simply the composite consequences of the deeds of other lives. We have no one to thank but ourselves. It is no use trying to bargain with Iswara, or propitiate Him, or hold Him responsible for our troubles. It is no use

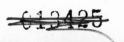

inventing a Devil as an alibi for our weakness. Maya is what we make of it—and Iswara simply represents that stern and solemn fact.

Viewed from a relative standpoint, this world of appearance is a bleak place, and as such it often drives us to despair. The seers, with their larger knowledge, tell us otherwise. Once we become conscious, even dimly, of the Atman, the Reality within us, the world takes on a very different aspect. It is no longer a court of justice but a kind of gymnasium. Good and evil, pain and pleasure, still exist, but they seem more like the ropes and vaulting-horses and parallel bars which can be used to make our bodies strong. Maya is no longer an endlessly revolving wheel of pain and pleasure but a ladder which can be climbed to consciousness of the Reality. From this stand-point, fortune and misfortune are both "mercies" —that is to say, opportunities. Every experience offers us the chance of making a constructive reaction to it—a reaction which helps to break some chain of our bondage to Maya and bring us that much nearer to spiritual freedom. Shankara therefore distinguishes between two kinds of Maya—avidya (evil or ignorance) and vidya (good). Avidya is that which causes us to move further away from the real Self, and veils our knowledge of the Truth. Vidya is that which enables us to come nearer to the real Self by removing the veil of ignorance. Both vidya and avidya are transcended when we pass beyond Maya into consciousness of the absolute Reality.

It has been said already that the principle of Maya is the superimposition of the ego-idea upon the Atman, the real Self. The ego-idea represents a false claim to individuality, to being different from our neighbors. It follows, therefore, that any act which contradicts this claim will bring us one step back toward right knowledge, to consciousness of the inner Reality. If we recognize our brotherhood with our fellow-men; if we try to deal honestly, truthfully, charitably with them; if, politically and economically, we work for equal rights, equal justice and the abolition of barriers of race and class and creed, then we are in fact giving the lie to the ego-idea and moving toward awareness of the universal, non-individual Existence. All such actions and motives belong to what is known as ethical goodness—just as all selfish motives and actions belong to ethical evil. In this sense, and in this sense only, goodness may be said to be more "real", or more valid, than evil—since evil actions and thoughts involve us more deeply in Maya, while good thoughts and actions lead us beyond Maya, to consciousness of the Reality.

The words "sin" and "virtue" are somewhat alien to the spirit of Vedanta Philosophy, because they necessarily foster a sense of possessiveness with regard to thought and action. If we say "I am good" or "I am bad", we are only talking the language of Maya. "I am Brahman" is the only true statement any of us can make. St. François de Sales wrote that "even our repentance must be peaceful"—meaning that exaggerated remorse, just as much as excessive self-congratulation, simply binds us more firmly to the ego-idea, the lie of Maya. We must never forget that ethical conduct is a means, not an end in itself. Knowledge of the impersonal Reality is the only valid knowledge. Apart from that, our deepest wisdom is black ignorance and our strictest righteousness is all in vain.

## The Supreme Goal

It may be objected that Vedanta Philosophy, like every other system of religious thought, is based upon a central hypothesis. Certainly, the supreme goal of life is to know Brahman—if Brahman exists. But can we be sure of this? Isn't it possible that there is no underlying reality in the universe? Isn't it possible that life is just a meaningless flux, dying and becoming, in perpetual change?

What is so attractive about Vedanta is its undogmatic, experimental approach to truth. Shankara does not tell us that we must accept the existence of Brahman as a dogma before we can enter upon the spiritual life. No—he invites us to find out for ourselves.

Nothing—no teacher, no scripture—can do the work for us. Teachers and scriptures are merely encouragements to personal effort. But, as such, they can be very impressive. Imagine that this is a law-suit and that you are the judge. Try to listen impartially to the witnesses on both sides. Consider the witnesses for Brahman—the seers and saints who claim to have known the eternal Reality. Consider their personalities, their words, the circumstances of their lives. Ask yourself—are these men liars or hypocrites or insane, or are they telling the truth? Compare the great scriptures of the world and ask—do they contradict each other, or do they agree? Then give your verdict.

But mere assent, as Shankara insists, is not enough. It is only a preliminary step toward active participation in the search. Direct personal experience is the only satisfactory proof of Brahman's existence, and each of us must have it.

Modern science goes a long way toward confirming the Vedanta world-picture. It admits that consciousness, in varying degrees, may be present everywhere. Differences between objects and creatures are only surface-differences, varying arrangements of atoms. Elements can be changed into other elements. Identity is only provisional. Science does not yet accept the concept of absolute Reality, but it certainly does not exclude it. Shankara knew nothing of modern science, but his approach is fundamentally scientific. It is based upon the practice of discrimination—a discrimination to be applied to ourselves and to every circumstance and object of our experience, at each instant of our lives. Again and again— thousands and thousands of times a day—we must ask ourselves "is this real or unreal, is this fact or fancy, is this nature or only appearance?" Thus, we probe deeper and deeper toward the truth.

We all know that we exist. We are all aware of our own consciousness. But what is the nature of this consciousness, this existence? Discrimination will soon prove to us that the ego-idea is not the fundamental reality. There is something beyond it. We can call this something "Brahman"—but Brahman is only another word. It does not reveal the nature of the thing we are looking for.

*Can* Brahman be known as an existing substance or thing? Not in the ordinary meaning of the verb. To know something is to obtain objective knowledge of it, and such knowledge is relative, depending upon space, time and causation. We cannot know absolute consciousness in this manner, because absolute consciousness is knowledge itself. Brahman is the source of all other knowledge; it comprises the knower, the knowledge and that which is known. It is independent of space, time and cause.

In this sense, the practice of discrimination differs from the method of scientific research. The scientist concentrates upon some object of knowledge, and pursues it beyond the range of physical sense-perception, with the aid of apparatus, chemical analysis, mathematics and so forth. His research extends like a journey, deeper and deeper into time and space. The religious philosopher is trying to annihilate time and space, the dimensions of the ego-idea, and thus uncover the Reality which is nearer and more instant than the ego, the body or the mind.

He is trying to be aware of what he already and always is—and this awareness is not an aspect of consciousness itself. The illumined seer does not merely know Brahman; he *is* Brahman, he *is* Existence, he *is* Knowledge. Absolute freedom is not something to be attained, absolute knowledge is not something to be gained, Brahman is not something to be found. It is only Maya which has to be pierced, ignorance which has to be overcome. The process of discrimination is a negative process. The positive fact, our real nature, eternally exists. We *are* Brahman—and only ignorance divides us from this knowledge.

Transcendental consciousness, or union with Brahman, can never be investigated by the methods of scientific research, since such research depends ultimately upon sense-perception, and Brahman is beyond the grasp of the senses. But this does not mean that we are doomed to doubt—or to blind trust in the experience of the seers—until we have reached the Supreme Goal for ourselves. Even a little effort in meditation and the spiritual life will reward us with insight and conviction that this is really the way to truth and peace—that we are not simply deceiving or hypnotizing ourselves—that Reality *is* available. We shall have our ups and downs, of course, and our moments of uncertainty, but we shall always return to this conviction. No spiritual gain, however small, is ever lost or wasted.

## Methods and Means

There are many paths to the attainment of transcendental consciousness. In Sanskrit, these paths are called Yogas, or ways to union with Brahman. Different Yogas suit different temperaments. Indeed, each individual will approach the Reality in a slightly different manner.

Four main Yogas are generally recognized in Hindu religious literature—Karma, Bhakti, Jnana and Raja. Very briefly, their characteristics are as follows:

Karma Yoga, as its name implies, is concerned

with work and action. By working selflessly for our neighbors, by regarding all action as a sacramental offering to God, by doing our duty without anxiety or concern for success or failure, praise or blame, we can gradually annihilate the ego-idea. Through Karma we can transcend Karma and experience the Reality which is beyond all action.

Bhakti is the Yoga of devotion—devotion to Iswara, the Personal God, or to a great teacher, a Christ, a Buddha, a Ramakrishna. Through this personal devotion, this loving service to an embodied ideal, the devotee will ultimately transcend personality altogether. This is the Yoga of ritual, of worship, of the religious sacraments. Ritual plays an important part in it, as a physical aid to concentration—for the acts of ritual, like the acts of Karma Yoga, bring the mind back repeatedly from its distractions and help to keep it steadily upon its object. For many, it is the easiest path to follow.

Jnana Yoga, on the other hand, is more suited to those whose powerful and austere intellects mistrust the emotional fervour of worship. It is the Yoga of pure discrimination. It transcends the intellect through the intellect. It needs no Iswara, no altar, no image, no ritual. It seeks a more immediate approach to the Impersonal Brahman. This path may perhaps be more direct, but it is also hard and steep, and can be trodden only by a few.

Raja Yoga—the Yoga of meditation—combines, to some extent, the three others. It does not exclude Karma Yoga, and it makes use both of the

Bhakti and the Jnana approach—since true meditation is a blend of the devotional and the discriminative.

By temperament, Shankara inclined toward Jnana Yoga, the way of pure discrimination—although, as this book will show, he was capable of great devotion also. Renunciation, discrimination, self-control—these are his watchwords. Some may find his austerity too forbidding, especially in the earlier portion of the dialogue; but it is precisely this severity which supplies a valuable corrective to the dangers of an easy sentimentality, an excess of carefree optimism, a confusion of real devotion with mere emotional self-indulgence. Shankara was under no illusions about this world of Maya; he condemns its apparent pleasures and delights with brutal frankness. For this very reason he was able to describe so powerfully the complete transformation of the universe which takes place before the eyes of the illumined seer. When Brahman is experienced, when all creatures and objects are seen in their real relation to the Absolute, then this world is indeed a paradise; it is nothing but Brahman, nothing but utter consciousness, knowledge and peace. After arduous struggles, the pupil in the "Crest Jewel" achieves this realization, and Shankara's book closes with the magnificent outburst of his joy.

# III

SHANKARA'S

# Crest-Jewel of Discrimination

*(Viveka-Chudamani)*

I PROSTRATE myself before Govinda, the perfect teacher, who is absorbed always in the highest state of bliss. His true nature cannot be known by the senses or the mind. It is revealed only through knowledge of the scriptures.

## The Path

IT IS hard for any living creature to achieve birth in a human form. Strength of body and will are even harder to obtain; purity is harder still; harder even than these is the desire to live a spiritual life; and an understanding of the scriptures is hardest of all. As for discrimination between the Atman and the non-Atman, direct perception of the

Atman itself, continuous union with Brahman, and final liberation—these cannot be obtained except through the merits of a hundred billion well-lived incarnations.

Only through God's grace may we obtain those three rarest advantages—human birth, the longing for liberation, and discipleship to an illumined teacher.

Nevertheless, there are those who somehow manage to obtain this rare human birth, together with bodily and mental strength, and an understanding of the scriptures—and yet are so deluded that they do not struggle for liberation. Such men are suicides. They clutch at the unreal and destroy themselves.

For what greater fool can there be than the man who has obtained this rare human birth together with bodily and mental strength and yet fails, through delusion, to realize his own highest good?

Men may recite the scriptures and sacrifice to the holy spirits, they may perform rituals and worship deities—but, until a man wakes to knowledge of his identity with the Atman, liberation can never be obtained; no, not even at the end of many hundreds of ages.

The scriptures declare that immortality cannot be gained through work or progeny or riches, but by renunciation alone. Hence it is clear that work cannot bring us liberation.

Therefore, let the wise man give up craving for pleasure in external things, and struggle hard for liberation. Let him seek out a noble and high-souled teacher, and become absorbed wholeheartedly in the truth which is taught him.

Through devotion to right discrimination he will climb to the height of union with Brahman. By the power of the Atman, let him rescue his own soul which lies drowned in the vast waters of worldliness.

Let the wise, who have grown tranquil and who practice contemplation of the Atman, give up all worldly activities and struggle to cut the bonds of worldliness.

Right action helps to purify the heart, but it does not give us direct perception of the Reality. The Reality is attained through discrimination, but not in the smallest degree by ten million acts.

Correct discernment shows us the true nature of a rope, and removes the painful fear caused by our deluded belief that it is a large snake.

Certain knowledge of the Reality is gained only through meditation upon right teaching, and not by sacred ablutions, or almsgiving, or by the practice of hundreds of breathing exercises.

Success in attaining the goal depends chiefly upon the qualifications of the seeker. Suitable time, place and other such circumstances are aids to its attainment.

Therefore, let him who would know the Atman which is the Reality practice discrimination. But first he must approach a teacher who is a perfect knower of Brahman, and whose compassion is as vast as the ocean itself.

## The Disciple

A MAN should be intelligent and learned, with great powers of comprehension, and able to overcome doubts by the exercise of his reason. One who has these qualifications is fitted for knowledge of the Atman.

He alone may be considered qualified to seek Brahman who has discrimination, whose mind is turned away from all enjoyments, who possesses tranquillity and the kindred virtues, and who feels a longing for liberation.

In this connection, the sages have spoken of four qualifications for attainment. When these are present, devotion to the Reality will become complete. When they are absent, it will fail.

First is mentioned discrimination between the eternal and the non-eternal. Next comes renunciation of the enjoyment of the fruits of action, here and hereafter. Then come the six treasures of virtue, beginning with tranquillity. And last, certainly, is the longing for liberation.

Brahman is real; the universe is unreal. A firm conviction that this is so is called *discrimination* between the eternal and the non-eternal.

*Renunciation* is the giving-up of all the pleasures of the eyes, the ears, and the other senses, the giving-up of all objects of transitory enjoyment, the giving-up of the desire for a physical body as well as for the highest kind of spirit-body of a god.

To detach the mind from all objective things by continually seeing their imperfection, and to direct it steadfastly toward Brahman, its goal—this is called *tranquillity*.

To detach both kinds of sense-organs—those of perception and those of action—from objective things, and to withdraw them to rest in their respective centers—this is called *self-control*. True *mental poise*, consists in not letting the mind react to external stimuli.

To endure all kinds of afflictions without rebellion, complaint or lament—this is called *forbearance*.

A firm conviction, based upon intellectual understanding that the teachings of the scriptures and of one's master are true—this is called by the sages the *faith* which leads to realization of the Reality.

To concentrate the intellect repeatedly upon the pure Brahman and to keep it fixed there always—this is called *self-surrender*. This does not mean soothing the mind, like a baby, with idle thoughts.

*Longing for liberation* is the will to be free from the fetters forged by ignorance—beginning with the ego-sense and so on, down to the physical body itself—through the realization of one's true nature.

Even though this longing for liberation may be present in a slight or moderate degree, it will grow intense through the grace of the teacher, and through the practice of renunciation and of virtues such as tranquillity, etc.: And it will bear fruit.

When renunciation and the longing for liberation are present to an intense degree within a man, then the practice of tranquillity and the other virtues will bear fruit and lead to the goal.

Where renunciation and longing for liberation are weak, tranquillity and the other virtues are a mere appearance, like the mirage in the desert.

Among all means of liberation, devotion is supreme. To seek earnestly to know one's real nature—this is said to be devotion.

In other words, devotion can be defined as the search for the reality of one's own Atman. The seeker after the reality of the Atman, who possesses the above-mentioned qualifications, should approach an illumined teacher from whom he can learn the way to liberation from all bondage.

## The Teacher

A TEACHER is one who is deeply versed in the scriptures, pure, free from lust, a perfect knower of Brahman. He is upheld continually in Brahman, calm like the flame when its fuel is consumed, an ocean of the love that knows no ulterior motive, a friend to all good people who humbly entrust themselves to him.

Let the seeker approach the master with reverent devotion. Then, when he has pleased him by his humility, love and service, let him ask whatever may be known about the Atman.

O Master, friend of all devotees, I bow down before you. O boundless compassion, I have fallen into the sea of the world—save me with those steadfast eyes which shed grace, like nectar, never-ending.

I am burning in the blaze of the world-forest, which no man can extinguish. Evil deeds out of the past drive me like huge winds, hither and thither. I am full of fear. I have taken refuge in you. Save me from death. I know no other shelter.

There are pure souls who have attained peace and greatness. They bring good to mankind, like the coming of spring. They themselves have crossed the dreadful ocean of this world. Without any selfish motive, they help others to cross.

It is the very nature of these great souls to work, of their own accord, to cure the troubles of others; just as the moon, of its own accord, cools the earth when it is scorched by the fierce rays of the sun.

The vessel of your lips has been dipped in and filled with the sweetness of the bliss of Brahman. Pour words from it like drops of nectar upon me. They are purifying, soothing and delightful to the ear. Master, I am consumed by the scorching heat of this worldly life, as by the flames of a forest-fire. Blessed are they on whom your eye rests even for a moment—it is thus that you accept them and make them your own.

How shall I cross the ocean of this world? What should be my goal? What way should I take? I know of none. Be gracious, Master. Save me. Tell me how to end the miseries of this earthly life. Withhold nothing.

Scorched by the fierce flames of the world-forest, the disciple speaks these words. The great soul looks at the disciple who thus seeks refuge in him, and his eyes are wet with tears of mercy. Immediately, he frees the disciple from his fear.

This disciple, who has sought his protection, is one who thirsts for liberation, who has properly fulfilled his duties, whose heart has become tranquil and who has attained calmness of mind. The wise and holy man, out of compassion, begins to instruct him in the truth.

ॐ ॐ ॐ

O PRUDENT one, do not fear! For you there is no danger. There *is* a way to cross the ocean of worldly life. I shall reveal to you that very method by which sages have reached the other shore.

There is a certain potent method of putting an end to the horror of this worldly life. By it, you may cross the world-ocean and reach the highest bliss.

Meditation on the meaning of the truth as it is taught in Vedanta leads to the highest illumination. By this means, the misery of worldly life is altogether destroyed.

Faith, devotion, and constant union with God through prayer—these are declared by the sacred scriptures to be the seeker's direct means of liberation. To him who abides by them comes liberation from that bondage of physical consciousness which has been forged by ignorance.

Because you are associated with ignorance, the supreme Atman within you appears to be in bondage to the non-Atman. This is the sole cause of the cycle of births and deaths. The flame of illumination, which is kindled by discrimination between Atman and non-Atman, will burn away the effects of ignorance, down to their very roots.

## The Questions

*The Disciple speaks:*

Master, please listen to the questions I am about to ask. I shall feel blessed if I may hear an answer from your lips.

What, in reality, is this bondage? How did it begin? In what is it rooted? How is a man set free from it? What is the non-Atman? What is the

40

supreme Atman? How can one discriminate between them? Please answer me.

~ ~ ~

*The Master speaks:*

You are blessed indeed! You are drawing near
to the goal. Through you, your whole family has
become purified, because you long to get free
from the bondage of ignorance and reach Brahman.

Children may free their father from his debts,
but no other person can free a man from his
bondage: he must do it himself.

Others may relieve the suffering caused by a
burden that weighs upon the head; but the suffering which comes from hunger and the like can
only be relieved by one's self.

The sick man who takes medicine and follows
the rules of diet is seen to be restored to health—
but not through the efforts of another.

A clear vision of the Reality may be obtained
only through our own eyes, when they have been
opened by spiritual insight—never through the
eyes of some other seer. Through our own eyes
we learn what the moon looks like: how could
we learn this through the eyes of others?

Those cords that bind us, because of our ignorance, our lustful desires and the fruits of our
karma—how could anybody but ourselves untie
them, even in the course of innumerable ages?

Neither by the practice of Yoga or of Sankhya
philosophy, nor by good works, nor by learning,
does liberation come; but only through a realiza-

tion that Atman and Brahman are one—in no other way.

It is the duty of a king to please his people, but not everybody who pleases the people is fit to be a king. For the people can be pleased by the beauty of a vina's form, and the skill with which its strings are plucked.

Erudition, well-articulated speech, a wealth of words, and skill in expounding the scriptures— these things give pleasure to the learned, but they do not bring liberation.

Study of the scriptures is fruitless as long as Brahman has not been experienced. And when Brahman has been experienced, it is useless to read the scriptures.

A network of words is like a dense forest which causes the mind to wander hither and thither. Therefore, those who know this truth should struggle hard to experience Brahman.

When a man has been bitten by the snake of ignorance he can only be cured by the realization of Brahman. What use are Vedas or scriptures, charms or herbs?

A sickness is not cured by saying the word "medicine". You must take the medicine. Liberation does not come by merely saying the word "Brahman". Brahman must be actually experienced.

Until you allow this apparent universe to dissolve from your consciousness—until you have experienced Brahman—how can you find liberation just by saying the word "Brahman"? The result is merely a noise.

Until a man has destroyed his enemies and taken possession of the splendour and wealth of the kingdom, he cannot become a king by simply saying: "I am a king".

A buried treasure is not uncovered by merely uttering the words "come forth". You must follow the right directions, dig, remove the stones and earth from above it, and then make it your own. In the same way, the pure truth of the Atman, which is buried under Maya and the effects of Maya, can be reached by meditation, contemplation and other spiritual disciplines such as a knower of Brahman may prescribe—but never by subtle arguments.

Therefore the wise must personally exert all their powers to get liberation from the bondage of the world, just as they would personally take remedies against physical ailments.

♪ ♪ ♪

THE question you have asked today is a very good one. It is relevant to the teachings of the scriptures. Its meaning is hidden deep, as within an aphorism. It should be asked by all who seek liberation.

Listen attentively, O prudent one, to what I say. By listening, you shall certainly be liberated from the bonds of the world.

Of the steps to liberation, the first is declared to be complete detachment from all things which are non-eternal. Then comes the practice of tranquillity, self-control, and forbearance. And then the entire giving-up of all actions which are done from personal, selfish desire.

Then the disciple must hear the truth of the Atman, and reflect on it, and meditate upon it constantly, without pause, for a long time. Thus the wise man reaches that highest state, in which consciousness of subject and object is dissolved away and the infinite unitary consciousness alone remains—and he knows the bliss of Nirvana while still living on earth.

## Atman and Non-Atman

NOW I shall explain discrimination between the Atman and the non-Atman, which you must learn. Listen carefully; then realize the truth of it within your own soul.

What the seers call the gross body is made up of these substances—marrow, bone, fat, flesh, blood, skin, and epidermis. It consists of legs, thighs, chest, arms, feet, back, head, and other parts. It is known to be the root of that delusion of "I" and "mine".

The subtle elements are ether, air, fire, water and earth. Portions of each of these, compounded together, compose the gross body.

Sound, touch, sight, taste and smell—these five essences of the elements are what we experience. They exist in order to be experienced by the individual man.

Those deluded beings who are tied to the objects they experience by the strong cord of desire, so hard to break, remain subject to birth and death. They travel upward or downward, impelled by their own karma, that inescapable law.

The deer, the elephant, the moth, the fish and the bee—each of these goes to its death under the fascination of one single sense out of the five. What, then, must be the fate that awaits a man who is under the fascination of all five senses?

The objects experienced by the senses are even stronger in their evil effects than the poison of the cobra. Poison kills only when it is absorbed into the body, but these objects destroy us merely by being seen with the eyes.

Only he who is free from the horrible trap of craving for sense-enjoyment, so hard to renounce, is ready for liberation—and no other, even though he may be schooled in the six systems of philosophy.

So-called seekers for liberation, who lack the true spirit of renunciation, try, nevertheless, to cross the ocean of this world. The shark of craving catches them by the throat, and drags them violently from their course, and they are drowned mid-way.

He who has killed the shark of sense-craving with the sword of true dispassion, crosses the ocean of this world without meeting any obstacle.

Know that that deluded man who walks the dreadful path of sense-craving, moves nearer to his ruin with every step. And know this to be true also—that he who walks the path indicated by his teacher, who is his truest well-wisher, and by his own better judgement, reaps the highest fruit of the knowledge of Brahman.

If you really desire liberation, hold the objects of sense-enjoyment at a distance, like poison; and keep drinking in with delight such virtues as contentment, compassion, forgiveness, straightforwardness, tranquillity and self-control, as if they were nectar.

A man should be continually occupied in trying to free himself from the bondage of ignorance, which is without beginning. He who neglects this duty and is passionately absorbed in feeding the cravings of the body, commits suicide thereby. For the body is merely a vehicle of experience for the human spirit.

He who tries to find the Atman by feeding the cravings of the body, is trying to cross a river by grasping a crocodile, mistaking it for a log.

Attachment to body, objects and persons is considered fatal to a seeker for liberation. He who has completely overcome attachment is ready for the state of liberation.

Kill this deadly attachment to body, wife, children and others. The seers who have overcome it go to that high dwelling-place of Vishnu, the all-pervading.

This body, which is made up of skin, flesh, blood, arteries, veins, fat, marrow and bone, is full of waste matter and filth. It deserves our contempt.

## Waking, Dreaming, Dreamless Sleep

THIS physical body is composed of the gross elements, which are formed by a five-fold compound of their subtle elements. It is born through the karma of the previous life, and is the vehicle of experience for the Atman. When the objective universe is being perceived, this is known as the waking state of consciousness.

In the waking state of consciousness, man finds his fullest activity in the body. In this state, he identifies himself with his body, although he is really separate from it. Through the external senses, he enjoys gross objects, such as garlands, perfumes, women and so forth, as well as other objects of sense-pleasure.

You must know that this body, through which man experiences the whole external world, is like the house of a householder.

The inherent characteristics of this gross body are birth, decay and death. It has various conditions, such as fatness or thinness; and various stages of development, such as childhood and youth. It is controlled by caste-rules, and the rules of the four orders of life. It is subject to various diseases, and to different kinds of treatment, such as worship, dishonor or honor.

Its organs of perception are the ears, skin, eyes, nose and tongue: through these we cognize objects. Its organs of action are the vocal organs, hands, legs, and the organs of excretion and reproduction. These involve us in action.

The mental organ consists of mind, intellect, ego, and the emotional nature. These are distinguished by their different functions. The function of mind is to consider the various aspects of an object. The function of the intellect is to determine the real nature of an object.

Ego is the self-consciousness which arises when the mental organ identifies itself with the body. The tendency of the emotional nature is to draw us to that which is pleasing.

The vital force is divided according to its five different functions. "Breath" is that function of the vital force which is used in respiration. "Downward breath" is used in excretion. "Distributive breath" governs the processes of digestion and assimilation. "Diffused breath" is present throughout the body, resisting disintegration, and holding it together in all its parts. "Ascending breath" is used in eructation. Just as gold is known by different names when it is fashioned into various ornaments, just as water takes the form of waves, foam, etc., so the one vital force is given these five different names according to its five different functions.

Eight groups make up the subtle body: Five organs of perception, five organs of action, five functions of the vital force, five subtle elements, and the mental organ, together with ignorance, desires and karma.

The subtle body is composed of the subtle elements before they have entered into their fivefold compounds. It is the seat of our desires. It is the field within which the fruits of karma are experienced. Because of human ignorance, this subtle body has been superimposed upon the Atman from time without beginning.

The dream-state belongs pre-eminently to the subtle body. In dreams, it creates its own kind of matter, and shines with its own light. The mental organ is the storehouse of the many impressions left by our desires in the waking-state. In dreams, the mental organ identifies itself with the sense of ego, and these impressions play over it. But the Atman remains beyond, as always, in its own self-luminous consciousness. At that time, the mental organ is its only covering. The Atman witnesses everything, but it is not in the least contaminated by our dream-experiences. It is free forever, and untouched. No karma created by its covering bodies can ever contaminate it, even to the smallest degree.

The subtle body is like a sharp tool in the hand of the carpenter. It is the instrument of the whole activity of the Atman, which is infinite wisdom. Therefore, the Atman itself is free from any taint.

The conditions of blindness, weakness and keen vision belong to the eye: they are caused by its qualities and defects. In the same way, deafness and dumbness are conditions of the ear and tongue—but not of the Atman, the knower.

Inhalation, exhalation, yawning, sneezing, the discharge of saliva, and the leaving of the body at death are said, by those who know, to be the various functions of the vital force. Hunger and thirst, also, are functions of the vital force.

The mental organ identifies itself with the organs of perception and of action, as well as with the physical body. Thus the sense of individuality arises, which causes a man to live and to act. His consciousness is a reflection of the infinite consciousness of the Atman.

He who believes himself to be acting or experiencing is known as the ego, the individual man. Identifying himself with the gunas, he experiences the three states of consciousness—waking, dreaming and dreamless sleep.

When the objects of experience are pleasant, he is happy. When they are unpleasant, he is unhappy. Pleasure and pain are characteristics of the individual—not of the Atman, which is forever blissful.

The object of experience is lovable—not for itself, but because it serves the Atman. But the

Atman itself is to be loved above all else. The Atman is forever blissful. For it, there can never be any suffering.

In dreamless sleep, when there is no object of experience, the joy of the Atman is felt. This is confirmed by our own experience—as well as by the scriptures, tradition, and logic.

## Maya

MAYA, in her potential aspect, is the divine power of the Lord. She has no beginning. She is composed of the three gunas, subtle, beyond perception. It is from the effects she produces that her existence is inferred by the wise. It is she who gives birth to the whole universe.

She is neither being nor non-being, nor a mixture of both. She is neither divided nor undivided, nor a mixture of both. She is neither an indivisible whole, nor composed of parts, nor a mixture of both. She is most strange. Her nature is inexplicable.

Just as knowing a rope to be a rope destroys the illusion that it is a snake, so Maya is destroyed by direct experience of Brahman—the pure, the free, the one without a second. Maya is composed of the gunas—the forces which are known as rajas, tamas and sattwa. These have distinctive characteristics.

Rajas has the power of projection: its nature is activity. Through its power, the phenomenal world, which is involved in Maya, begins to evolve. Attachment, desire and similar qualities are caused by its power, as are also grief and similar moods of the mind.

Lust, anger, greed, arrogance, jealousy, egotism, envy and other such vices are the worst characteristics of rajas. When a man is overpowered by it, he attaches himself to worldly actions. Hence rajas is the cause of bondage.

Tamas has the power of veiling the real nature of an object, making it appear other than it is. It is the cause of man's continued subjection to the wheel of birth and death. It also makes possible the operation of the power of rajas.

A man may be intelligent, clever, and learned. He may have the faculty of keen self-analysis. But, if he is overpowered by tamas, he cannot understand the true nature of the Atman, even thought it may be clearly explained to him in various ways. He takes the appearance, which is the product of his ignorance, for the reality—and so he becomes attached to delusions. This obscuring power of dreadful tamas is, alas, very great.

Failure to perceive the actual object, seeing something as different from what it really is, vacillation of the mind, taking delusions for realities: these are the characteristics of tamas. As long as a man is attached to tamas, he can never get free from them. And rajas, also, will trouble him without ceasing.

Tamas has these further characteristics: ignorance, laziness, dullness, sleep, delusion and stupidity. A man who is under their influence cannot understand anything. He lives like a somnambulist, or an unconscious log of wood.

Sattwa is purity. Even when it is mixed with rajas and tamas, as water is mixed with water, it lights the way to liberation. Sattwa reveals the Atman as the sun reveals the objective world.

Sattwa, when mixed with the other gunas, has these characteristics: absence of pride, purity, contentment, austerity, a desire to study the scriptures, self-surrender to God, harmlessness, truthfulness, continence, freedom from greed, faith, devotion, longing for liberation, aversion to the things of this world, and the other virtues that lead toward God.

Sattwa in its pure state has the following characteristics: tranquillity, direct perception of the Atman, absolute peace, contentment, joy and steady devotion to the Atman. Through these, the seeker tastes everlasting bliss.

Maya has been defined as a composition of the three gunas. It is the causal body of the Atman. Dreamless sleep belongs pre-eminently to the causal body. In this state, the workings of the mind and sense-organs are suspended.

In dreamless sleep, there is no cognition of any kind. But the mind continues to exist in its subtle form, like a seed. The proof of this can be found in everybody's experience—that the mind, when we wake up, still remembers: "I knew nothing."

There are the body, the sense-organs, the vital force, the mind, the ego and all their functions, the objects of enjoyment, pleasures and all other kinds of experience, the gross and the subtle elements—in short, the whole objective universe, and Maya which is its cause. None of these is the Atman.

You must know that Maya and all its effects—

from the cosmic intellect down to the gross body—are other than the Atman. All are unreal, like a mirage in the desert.

## The Atman

NOW I shall tell you the nature of the Atman. If you realize it, you will be freed from the bonds of ignorance, and attain liberation.

There is a self-existent Reality, which is the basis of our consciousness of ego. That Reality is the witness of the three states of our consciousness, and is distinct from the five bodily coverings.

That Reality is the knower in all states of consciousness—waking, dreaming and dreamless sleep. It is aware of the presence or absence of the mind and its functions. It is the Atman.

That Reality sees everything by its own light. No one sees it. It gives intelligence to the mind and the intellect, but no one gives it light.

That Reality pervades the universe, but no one penetrates it. It alone shines. The universe shines with its reflected light.

Because of its presence, the body, senses, mind and intellect apply themselves to their respective functions, as though obeying its command.

Its nature is eternal consciousness. It knows all things, from the sense of ego to the body itself. It is the knower of pleasure and pain and of the sense-objects. It knows everything objectively—just as a man knows the objective existence of a jar.

This is the Atman, the Supreme being, the ancient. It never ceases to experience infinite joy.

It is always the same. It is consciousness itself. The organs and vital energies function under its command.

Here, within this body, in the pure mind, in the secret chamber of intelligence, in the infinite universe within the heart, the Atman shines in its captivating splendour, like a noonday sun. By its light, the universe is revealed.

It is the knower of the activities of the mind and of the individual man. It is the witness of all the actions of the body, the sense-organs and the vital energy. It seems to be identified with all these, just as fire appears identified with an iron ball. But it neither acts nor is subject to the slightest change.

The Atman is birthless and deathless. It neither grows nor decays. It is unchangeable, eternal. It does not dissolve when the body dissolves. Does the ether cease to exist when the jar that enclosed it is broken?

The Atman is distinct from Maya, the primal cause, and from her effect, the universe. The nature of the Atman is pure consciousness. The Atman reveals this entire universe of mind and matter. It cannot be defined. In and through the various states of consciousness—the waking, the dreaming and the sleeping—it maintains our unbroken awareness of identity. It manifests itself as the witness of the intelligence.

## The Mind

WITH a controlled mind and an intellect which is made pure and tranquil, you must realize the Atman directly, within yourself. Know the Atman as the real I. Thus you cross the shoreless ocean of worldliness, whose waves are birth and death. Live always in the knowledge of identity with Brahman, and be blessed.

Man is in bondage because he mistakes what is non-Atman for his real Self. This is caused by ignorance. Hence follows the misery of birth and death. Through ignorance, man identifies the Atman with the body, taking the perishable for the real. Therefore he nourishes this body, and anoints it, and guards it carefully. He becomes enmeshed in the things of the senses like a caterpillar in the threads of its cocoon.

Deluded by his ignorance, a man mistakes one thing for another. Lack of discernment will cause a man to think that a snake is a piece of rope. When he grasps it in this belief he runs a great risk. The acceptance of the unreal as real constitutes the state of bondage. Pay heed to this, my friend.

The Atman is indivisible, eternal, one without a second. It is eternally made manifest by the power of its own knowledge. Its glories are infinite. The veil of tamas hides the true nature of the Atman, just as an eclipse hides the rays of the sun.

When the pure rays of the Atman are thus concealed, the deluded man identifies himself with his body, which is non-Atman. Then rajas, which has the power of projecting illusory forms, afflicts him sorely. It binds him with chains of lust, anger and the other passions.

His mind becomes perverted. His consciousness of the Atman is swallowed up by the shark of total ignorance. Yeilding to the power of rajas, he identifies himself with the many motions and changes of the mind. Therefore he is swept hither and thither, now rising, now sinking, in the boundless ocean of birth and death, whose waters are full of the poison of sense-objects. This is indeed a miserable fate.

The sun's rays bring forth layers of cloud. By them, the sun is concealed; and so it appears that the clouds alone exist. In the same way, the ego, which is brought forth by the Atman, hides the true nature of the Atman; and so it appears that the ego alone exists.

On a stormy day the sun is swallowed up by thick clouds; and these clouds are attacked by sharp, chill blasts of wind. So, when the Atman is enveloped in the thick darkness of tamas, the terrible power of rajas attacks the deluded man with all kinds of sorrows.

Man's bondage is caused by the power of these two—tamas and rajas. Deluded by these, he mistakes the body for the Atman and strays on to the path that leads to death and rebirth.

Man's life in this relative world may be compared to a tree. Tamas is the seed. Identification of the Atman with the body is its sprouting forth. The cravings are its leaves. Work is its sap. The body is its trunk. The vital forces are its branches. The sense-organs are its twigs. The sense-objects are its flowers. Its fruits are the sufferings caused by various actions. The individual man is the bird who eats the fruit of the tree of life.

The Atman's bondage to the non-Atman springs from ignorance. It has no external cause.

It is said to be beginningless. It will continue indefinitely until a man becomes enlightened. As long as a man remains in this bondage it subjects him to a long train of miseries—birth, death, sickness, decrepitude, and so forth.

This bondage cannot be broken by weapons, or by wind, or by fire, or by millions of acts. Nothing but the sharp sword of knowledge can cut through this bondage. It is forged by discrimination and made keen by purity of heart, through divine grace.

A man must faithfully and devotedly fulfill the duties of life as the scriptures prescribe. This purifies his heart. A man whose heart is pure realizes the supreme Atman. Thereby he destroys his bondage to the world, root and all.

Wrapped in its five coverings, beginning with the physical, which are the products of its own Maya, the Atman remains hidden, as the water of a pond is hidden by a veil of scum.

When the scum is removed, the pure water is clearly seen. It takes away a man's thirst, cools him immediately and makes him happy.

When all the five coverings are removed, the pure Atman is revealed. It is revealed as God dwelling within; as unending, unalloyed bliss; as the supreme and self-luminous Being.

The wise man who seeks liberation from bondage must discriminate between Atman and non-Atman. In this way, he can realize the Atman, which is Infinite Being, Infinite Wisdom and Infinite Love. Thus he finds happiness.

The Atman dwells within, free from attachment and beyond all action. A man must separate this

Atman from every object of experience, as a stalk of grass is separated from its enveloping sheath. Then he must dissolve into the Atman all those appearances which make up the world of name and form. He is indeed a free soul who can remain thus absorbed in the Atman alone.

## The Body

THIS body is the "physical covering". Food made its birth possible; on food it lives; without food it must die. It consists of cuticle, skin, flesh, blood, bone and water. It cannot be the Atman, the ever-pure, the self-existent.

It did not exist before birth, it will not exist after death. It exists for a short while only, in the interim between them. Its very nature is transient, and subject to change. It is a compound, not an element. Its vitality is only a reflection. It is a sense-object, which can be perceived, like a jar. How can it be the Atman—the experiencer of all experiences?

The body consists of arms, legs and other limbs. It is not the Atman—for when some of these limbs have been cut off, a man may continue to live and function through his remaining organs. The body is controlled by another. It cannot be the Atman, the controller.

The Atman watches the body, with its various characteristics, actions and states of growth. That this Atman, which is the abiding reality, is of another nature than the body, must be self-evident.

The body is a bundle of bones held together by

flesh. It is very dirty and full of filth. The body can never be the same as the self-existent Atman, the knower. The nature of the Atman is quite different from that of the body.

It is the ignorant man who identifies himself with the body, which is compounded of skin, flesh, fat, bone and filth. The man of spiritual discrimination knows the Atman, his true being, the one supreme reality, as distinct from the body.

The fool thinks, "I am the body". The intelligent man thinks, "I am an individual soul united with the body". But the wise man, in the greatness of his knowledge and spiritual discrimination, sees the Atman as reality and thinks, "I am Brahman".

O fool, stop identifying yourself with this lump of skin, flesh, fat, bones and filth. Identify yourself with Brahman, the Absolute, the Atman in all beings. That is how you can attain the supreme peace.

The intelligent man may be learned in Vedanta and the moral laws. But there is not the least hope of his liberation until he stops mistakenly identifying himself with the body and the sense-organs. This identification is caused by delusion.

You never identify yourself with the shadow cast by your body, or with its reflection, or with the body you see in a dream or in your imagination. Therefore you should not identify yourself with this living body, either.

Those who live in ignorance identify the body with the Atman. This ignorance is the root-cause of birth, death and rebirth. Therefore you must strive earnestly to destroy it. When your heart is free from this ignorance, there will no longer be any possibility of your rebirth. You will reach immortality.

᪥  ᪥  ᪥

THAT covering of the Atman which is called "the vital covering" is made up of the vital force and the five organs of action. The body is called "the physical covering". It comes to life when it is enveloped by the vital covering. It is thus that the body engages in action.

This vital covering is not the Atman—for it is merely composed of the vital airs. Air-like, it enters and leaves the body. It does not know what is good or bad for itself, or for others. It is always dependent upon the Atman.

## Purification

THE mind, together with the organs of perception, forms the "mental covering". It causes the sense of "I" and "mine". It also causes us to discern objects. It is endowed with the power and faculty of differentiating objects by giving them various names. It is manifest, enveloping the "vital covering".

The mental covering may be compared to the sacrificial fire. It is fed by the fuel of many desires. The five organs of perception serve as priests. Objects of desire are poured upon it like a continous stream of oblations. Thus it is that this phenomenal universe is brought forth.

Ignorance is nowhere, except in the mind. The mind is filled with ignorance, and this causes the bondage of birth and death. When, in the enlightenment of the Atman, a man transcends the mind, the phenomenal universe disappears from him. When a man lives in the domain of mental ignorance, the phenomenal universe exists for him.

In dream, the mind is emptied of the objective universe, but it creates by its own power a complete universe of subject and object. The waking state is only a prolonged dream. The phenomenal universe exists in the mind.

In dreamless sleep, when the mind does not function, nothing exists. This is our universal experience. Man seems to be in bondage to birth and death. This is a fictitious creation of the mind, not a reality.

The wind collects the clouds, and the wind drives them away again. Mind creates bondage, and mind also removes bondage.

The mind creates attachment to the body and the things of this world. Thus it binds a man, as a beast is tied by a rope. But it is also the mind which creates in a man an utter distaste for sense-objects, as if for poison. Thus it frees him from his bondage.

The mind, therefore, is the cause of man's bondage and also of his liberation. It causes bondage when it is darkened by rajas. It causes liberation when it is freed from rajas and tamas, and made pure.

If discrimination and dispassion are practiced, to the exclusion of everything else, the mind will become pure and move toward liberation. Therefore the wise man who seeks liberation must develop both these qualities within himself.

That terrible tiger called an impure mind prowls in the forest of the sense-objects. The wise man who seeks liberation must not go there.

The mind of the experiencer creates all the objects which he experiences, while in the waking or the dreaming state. Ceaselessly, it creates the differences in men's bodies, color, social condition and race. It creates the variations of the gunas. It creates desires, actions and the fruits of actions.

Man is pure spirit, free from attachment. The mind deludes him. It binds him with the bonds of the body, the sense-organs and the life-breath. It creates in him the sense of "I" and "mine". It makes him wander endlessly among the fruits of the actions it has caused.

The error of identifying Atman with non-Atman is the cause of man's birth, death and rebirth. This false identification is created by the mind. Therefore, it is the mind that causes the misery of birth, death and rebirth for the man who has no discrimination and is tainted by rajas and tamas.

Therefore the wise, who know Reality, have declared that the mind is full of ignorance. Because of this ignorance, all the creatures of the universe are swept helplessly hither and thither, like masses of cloud before the wind.

Therefore, the seeker after liberation must work carefully to purify the mind. When the mind has been made pure, liberation is as easy to grasp as the fruit which lies in the palm of your hand.

Seek earnestly for liberation, and your lust for sense-objects will be rooted out. Practice detachment toward all actions. Have faith in the Reality. Devote yourself to the practice of spiritual disciplines, such as hearing the word of Brahman, reasoning and meditating upon it. Thus the mind will be freed from the evil of rajas.

The "mental covering", therefore, cannot be the Atman. It has a beginning and an end, and is subject to change. It is the abode of pain. It is an object of experience. The seer cannot be the thing which is seen.

## The Covering of Intellect

THE discriminating faculty with its powers of intelligence, together with the organs of perception, is known as the "covering of intellect". To be the doer is its distinguishing characteristic. It is the cause of man's birth, death and rebirth.

The power of intelligence that is in the "covering of intellect" is a reflection of the Atman, the pure consciousness. The "covering of intellect" is an effect of Maya. It possesses the faculty of knowing and acting. It always identifies itself entirely with the body, sense-organs, etc.

It has no beginning. It is characterized by its sense of ego. It constitutes the individual man. It is the initiator of all actions and undertakings. Impelled by the tendencies and impressions formed in previous births, it performs virtuous or sinful actions and experiences their results.

It gathers experiences by wandering through

many wombs of higher or lower degree. The states of waking and dreaming belong to this "covering of intellect". It experiences joy and sorrow.

Because of its sense of "I" and "mine", it constantly identifies itself with the body, and the physical states, and with the duties pertaining to the different stages and orders of life. This "covering of intellect" shines with a bright light because of its proximity to the shining Atman. It is a garment of the Atman, but man identifies himself with it and wanders around the circle of birth, death and rebirth because of his delusion.

The Atman, which is pure consciousness, is the light that shines in the shrine of the heart, the center of all vital force. It is immutable, but it becomes the "doer" and "experiencer" when it is mistakenly identified with the "covering of intellect".

The Atman assumes the limitations of the "covering of intellect" because it is mistakenly identified with that covering, which is totally different from itself. This man, who is the Atman, regards himself as being separate from it, and from Brahman, who is the one Atman in all creatures. An ignorant man, likewise, may regard a jar as being different from the clay of which it was made.

By its nature, the Atman is forever unchanging and perfect. But it assumes the character and nature of its coverings because it is mistakenly identified with them. Although fire is formless, it will assume the form of red-hot iron.

# Delusion

*The Disciple:*

Either because of delusion, or for some other reason, the Atman appears to be the individual self. This mistaken identification had no beginning; and that which had no beginning cannot have an end, either.

Therefore this mistake about the individual soul's identity must be eternal, and its wanderings through birth, death and rebirth must continue forever. Then how can there be any liberation? Master, kindly explain this to me.

ᔕ   ᔕ   ᔕ

*The Master:*

Your question is to the point, O prudent one. Listen to me attentively. Something which has been conjured up by delusion and only exists in your imagination, can never be accepted as a fact.

By its nature, the Atman is forever unattached, beyond action and formless. Its identity with objects is imaginary, not real. We say "the sky is blue". Has the sky any color?

The Atman is the witness—beyond all attributes, beyond action. It can be directly realized as pure consciousness and infinite bliss. Its appearance as an individual soul is caused by the delusion of our understanding, and has no reality. By its very nature, this appearance is unreal. When our delusion has been removed, it ceases to exist.

Its appearance as an individual soul lasts only as long as our delusion lasts; since this misapprehension arises from a delusion of our understanding. As long as our delusion continues, the rope appears to be a snake. When the delusion ends, the snake ceases to exist.

It is true that ignorance and its effects have existed from a time without any beginning. But ignorance, although beginningless, comes to an end when knowledge dawns. It is completely destroyed, root and all, like the dreams that vanish utterly when we wake. When something which was previously non-existent comes into being, this implies that it has been non-existent from a beginningless time. But this non-existence, although beginningless, ceases as soon as that thing comes into existence. It is clear, therefore, that ignorance, although beginningless, is not eternal.

We see that a previous state of non-existence may come to an end, even though it is beginningless. It is the same with the semblance of an individual self. This semblance is due to a false identification of the Atman with the intellect and the other coverings. The Atman, by its very nature, is essentially distinct and separate from them. The identification of the Atman with the intellect, etc., is caused by ignorance.

This false identification can be dispelled only by perfect knowledge. Perfect knowledge, according to the revealed scriptures, is the realization of the Atman as one with Brahman.

This is attained by an absolute discrimination between the Atman and the non-Atman. Therefore a man should practice discrimination between the Atman and the individual self.

Just as very muddy water shines transparently when the mud clears away, so the Atman shines with a pure lustre when the impurities have been removed.

When the darkness of unreality vanishes, the eternal Atman is clearly revealed. Therefore a man should strive to free the eternal Atman from the unrealities of egotism and delusion.

✍   ✍   ✍

THE "covering of intellect", which we have been discussing, cannot be the Atman—for the following reasons: it undergoes change; intelligence is not its inherent nature; it is finite; it is an object of experience; it is transitory. The non-eternal cannot, therefore, be the eternal Atman.

## The Covering of Bliss

THE "covering of bliss"[1] is that covering of the Atman which catches a reflection of the blissful Atman itself. Nevertheless, this covering is a creation of our ignorance. Its nature consists of the various degrees of happiness which are experienced when a desired object is gained. Its blissful nature is spontaneously felt by righteous men when they reap the reward of their good deeds. It expresses that joy which all living beings may experience without making any effort towards it.

The "covering of bliss" is fully revealed to us in the state of deep sleep. It is partially revealed in the waking and the dreaming states, when any desirable object is being enjoyed.

[1]Refers to the ego-idea in man.

This "covering of bliss" cannot be the Atman, for the following reasons: it has limitations; it is an effect of Maya; its joyful nature is experienced as the result of good deeds; it is of the same kind as the other coverings, which are all products of Maya.

꩜   ꩜   ꩜

IF WE reason and meditate on the truth of the scriptures, transcending all the five coverings of ignorance, we realize the ultimate Existence—which is the Atman, the witness, the infinite consciousness.

The Atman is self-luminous, distinct from the five coverings. It is the witness of the three states of consciousness. It is existence, changeless, pure, ever-blissful. It is to be realized by the man of discrimination as the Atman within himself.

## Atman is Brahman

*The Disciple:*
Master, if we reject these five coverings as unreal, it seems to me that nothing remains but the void. How, then, can there be an existence which the wise man may realize as one with his Atman?

*The Master:*
That is a good question, O prudent one. Your argument is clever. Nevertheless, there must be an existence, a reality, which perceives the ego-sense and the coverings and is also aware of the void which is their absence. This reality by itself remains unperceived. Sharpen your discrimina-

tion that you may know this Atman, which is the knower.

He who experiences is conscious of himself. Without an experiencer, there can be no self-consciousness.

The Atman is its own witness, since it is conscious of itself. The Atman is no other than Brahman.

∽ ∽ ∽

THE Atman is pure consciousness, clearly manifest as underlying the states of waking, dreaming and dreamless sleep. It is inwardly experienced as unbroken consciousness, the consciousness that I am I. It is the unchanging witness that experiences the ego, the intellect and the rest, with their various forms and changes. It is realized within one's own heart as existence, knowledge and bliss absolute. Realize this Atman within the shrine of your own heart.

The fool sees the reflection of the sun in the water of a jar, and thinks it is the sun. Man in the ignorance of his delusion sees the reflection of Pure Consciousness upon the coverings, and mistakes it for the real I.

In order to look at the sun, you must turn away from the jar, the water, and the sun's reflection in the water. The wise know that these three are only revealed by the reflection of the self-luminous sun. They are not the sun itself.

The body, the covering of intellect, the reflection of consciousness upon it—none of these is the Atman. The Atman is the witness, infinite consciousness, revealer of all things but distinct from all, no matter whether they be gross or subtle. It is the eternal reality, omnipresent, all-pervading, the subtlest of all subtleties. It has neither inside nor outside. It is the real I, hidden in the shrine of the heart. Realize fully the truth of the Atman. Be free from evil and impurity, and you shall pass beyond death.

*ᔐ  ᔐ  ᔐ*

KNOW the Atman, transcend all sorrows, and reach the fountain of joy. Be illumined by this knowledge, and you have nothing to fear. If you wish to find liberation, there is no other way of breaking the bonds of rebirth.

What can break the bondage and misery of this world? The knowledge that the Atman is Brahman. Then it is that you realize Him who is one without a second, and who is the absolute bliss.

Realize Brahman, and there will be no more returning to this world—the home of all sorrows. You must realize absolutely that the Atman is Brahman.

Then you will win Brahman for ever. He is the truth. He is existence and knowledge. He is absolute. He is pure and self-existent. He is eternal, unending joy. He is none other than the Atman.

The Atman is one with Brahman: this is the highest truth. Brahman alone is real. There is none but He. When He is known as the supreme reality there is no other existence but Brahman.

# The Universe

BRAHMAN is the reality—the one existence, absolutely independent of human thought or idea. Because of the ignorance of our human minds, the universe seems to be composed of diverse forms. It is Brahman alone.

A jar made of clay is not other than clay. It is clay essentially. The form of the jar has no independent existence. What, then, is the jar? Merely an invented name!

The form of the jar can never be perceived apart from the clay. What, then, is the jar? An appearance! The reality is the clay itself.

This universe is an effect of Brahman. It can never be anything else but Brahman. Apart from Brahman, it does not exist. There is nothing beside Him. He who says that this universe has an independent existence is still suffering from delusion. He is like a man talking in his sleep.

"The universe is Brahman"—so says the great seer of the Atharva Veda. The universe, therefore, is nothing but Brahman. It is superimposed upon Him. It has no separate existence, apart from its ground.

If the universe, as we perceive it, were real, knowledge of the Atman would not put an end to our delusion. The scriptures would be untrue. The revelations of the Divine Incarnations would make no sense. These alternatives cannot be considered either desirable or beneficial by any thinking person.

Sri Krishna, the Incarnate Lord, who knows the secret of all truths, says in the Gita: "Although I am not within any creature, all creatures exist within me. I do not mean that they exist within me physically. That is my divine mystery. My Being sustains all creatures and brings them to birth, but has no physical contact with them."

If this universe were real, we should continue to perceive it in deep sleep. But we perceive nothing then. Therefore it is unreal, like our dreams.

The universe does not exist apart from the Atman. Our perception of it as having an independent existence is false, like our perception of blueness in the sky. How can a superimposed attribute have any existence, apart from its substratum? It is only our delusion which causes this misconception of the underlying reality.

No matter what a deluded man may think he is perceiving, he is really seeing Brahman and nothing else but Brahman. He sees mother-of-pearl and imagines that it is silver. He sees Brahman and imagines that it is the universe. But this universe, which is superimposed upon Brahman, is nothing but a name.

## I am Brahman

BRAHMAN is supreme. He is the reality—the one without a second. He is pure consciousness, free from any taint. He is tranquillity itself. He has neither beginning nor end. He does not change. He is joy for ever.

He transcends the appearance of the manifold, created by Maya. He is eternal, for ever beyond reach of pain, not to be divided, not to be measured, without form, without name, undifferentiated, immutable. He shines with His own light. He is everything that can be experienced in this universe.

The illumined seers know Him as the uttermost reality, infinite, absolute, without parts—the pure consciousness. In Him they find that knower, knowledge and known have become one.

They know Him as the reality which can neither be cast aside (since He is ever-present within the human soul) nor grasped (since He is beyond the power of mind and speech). They know Him immeasurable, beginningless, endless, supreme in glory. They realize the truth: "I am Brahman".

## That art Thou

THE scriptures establish the absolute identity of Atman and Brahman by declaring repeatedly: "That art Thou". The terms "Brahman" and "Atman", in their true meaning, refer to "That" and "Thou" respectively.

In their literal, superficial meaning, "Brahman" and "Atman" have opposite attributes, like the sun and the glow-worm, the king and his servant, the ocean and the well, or Mount Meru and the atom. Their identity is established only when they are understood in their true significance, and not in a superficial sense.

"Brahman" may refer to God, the ruler of Maya and creator of the universe. The "Atman" may refer to the individual soul, associated with the five coverings which are effects of Maya. Thus regarded, they possess opposite attributes. But this apparent opposition is caused by Maya and her effects. It is not real, therefore, but superimposed.

These attributes caused by Maya and her effects are superimposed upon God and upon the individual soul. When they have been completely eliminated, neither soul nor God remains. If you take the kingdom from a king and the weapons from a soldier, there is neither soldier nor king.

The scriptures repudiate any idea of a duality in Brahman. Let a man seek illumination in the knowledge of Brahman, as the scriptures direct. Then those attributes, which our ignorance has superimposed upon Brahman, will disappear.

"Brahman is neither the gross nor the subtle universe. The apparent world is caused by our imagination, in its ignorance. It is not real. It is like seeing the snake in the rope. It is like a passing dream"—that is how a man should practice spiritual discrimination, and free himself from his consciousness of this objective world. Then let him meditate upon the identity of Brahman and Atman, and so realize the truth.

Through spiritual discrimination, let him understand the true inner meaning of the terms "Brahman" and "Atman", thus realizing their absolute identity. See the reality in both, and you will find that there is but one.

When we say: "This man is that same Devadatta whom I have previously met", we establish a person's identity by disregarding those attributes superimposed upon him by the circumstances of our former meeting. In just the same way, when we consider the scriptural teaching "That art Thou", we must disregard those attributes which have been superimposed upon "That" and "Thou".

The wise men of true discrimination understand that the essence of both Brahman and Atman is Pure Consciousness, and thus realize their absolute identity. The identity of Brahman and Atman is declared in hundreds of holy texts.

Give up the false notion that the Atman is this body, this phantom. Meditate upon the truth that the Atman is "neither gross nor subtle, neither short nor tall", that it is self-existent, free as the sky, beyond the grasp of thought. Purify the heart until you know that "I am Brahman". Realize your own Atman, the pure and infinite consciousness.

Just as a clay jar or vessel is understood to be nothing but clay, so this whole universe, born of Brahman, essentially Brahman, is Brahman only—for there is nothing else but Brahman, nothing beyond That. That is the reality. That is our Atman. Therefore, "That art Thou"—pure, blissful, supreme Brahman, the one without a second.

You may dream of place, time, objects, individuals, and so forth. But they are unreal. In your waking state, you experience this world, but that experience arises from your ignorance. It is a prolonged dream, and therefore unreal. Unreal also are this body, these organs, this life-breath, this sense of ego. Therefore, "That art Thou"— pure, blissful, supreme Brahman, the one without a second.

Because of delusion, you may mistake one thing for another. But, when you know its real nature, then that nature alone exists, there is nothing else but that. When the dream breaks, the dream-universe has vanished. Does it appear, when you wake, that you are other than yourself?

Caste, creed, family and lineage do not exist in Brahman. Brahman has neither name nor form; it transcends merit and demerit; it is beyond time, space and the objects of sense-experience. Such is Brahman, and "That art Thou". Meditate upon this truth.

It is supreme. It is beyond the expression of speech; but it is known by the eye of pure illumination. It is pure, absolute consciousness, the eternal reality. Such is Brahman, and "That art Thou". Meditate upon this truth.

It is untouched by those six waves—hunger, thirst, grief, delusion, decay and death—which sweep the ocean of worldliness. He who seeks union with it must meditate upon it within the shrine of the heart. It is beyond the grasp of the senses. The intellect cannot understand it. It is out of the reach of thought. Such is Brahman, and "That art Thou". Meditate upon this truth.

It is the ground upon which this manifold universe, the creation of ignorance, appears to rest. It is its own support. It is neither the gross nor the subtle universe. It is indivisible. It is beyond comparison. Such is Brahman, and "That art Thou". Meditate upon this truth.

It is free from birth, growth, change, decline, sickness and death. It is eternal. It is the cause of the evolution of the universe, its preservation and its dissolution. Such is Brahman, and "That art Thou". Meditate upon this truth.

It knows no differentiation or death. It is calm, like a vast, waveless expanse of water. It is eternally free and indivisible. Such is Brahman, and "That art Thou". Meditate upon this truth.

Though one, it is the cause of the many. It is the one and only cause, no other beside it. It has no cause but itself. It is independent, also, of the law of causation. It stands alone. Such is Brahman, and "That art Thou". Meditate upon this truth.

It is unchangeable, infinite, imperishable. It is beyond Maya and her effects. It is eternal, undying bliss. It is pure. Such is Brahman, and "That art Thou". Meditate upon this truth.

It is that one Reality which appears to our ignorance as a manifold universe of names and forms and changes. Like the gold of which many ornaments are made, it remains in itself unchanged. Such is Brahman, and "That art Thou". Meditate upon this truth.

There is nothing beyond it. It is greater than the greatest. It is the innermost self, the ceaseless joy within us. It is absolute existence, knowledge and bliss. It is endless, eternal. Such is Brahman, and "That art Thou". Meditate upon this truth.

Meditate upon this truth, following the arguments of the scriptures by the aid of reason and intellect. Thus you will be freed from doubt and confusion, and realize the truth of Brahman. This truth will become as plain to you as water held in the palm of your hand.

# Devotion

As a king is recognized distinctly amidst his army, so realize Brahman as pure consciousness, distinct from all imperfections. Dwell for ever in the Atman. Let this manifest world melt away in Brahman.

Brahman dwells within the shrine of the heart—the eternal existence, the supreme, the one without a second, standing apart from the gross and subtle aspects of this universe. The man who dwells within this shrine, united with Brahman, is no longer subject to rebirth and death.

The truth of Brahman may be understood intellectually. But the ego-sense is deep-rooted and powerful, for it has existed from beginningless time. It creates the impression that "I am the actor, I am he who experiences". This impression causes our bondage to rebirth and death. It can be removed only by the earnest effort to live constantly in union with Brahman. The sages define liberation as freedom from all such impressions, and hence from the cravings which are caused by them.

It is ignorance that causes our sense of identity with the body, the sense-organs and everything else which is not the Atman. He is a wise man who overcomes this ignorance through devotion to the Atman.

Know your true Atman as the witness of the mind and intellect, and of the thought-waves that arise in them. Raise one single wave of thought constantly: "I am Brahman". Thus you will free yourself from identification with non-Atman.

CEASE to follow the way of the world, cease to follow the way of the flesh, cease to follow the way of tradition. Get rid of this false identification and know the true Atman.

When a man follows the way of the world, the way of tradition and the way of the flesh, knowledge of the Reality is not born within him.

The wise say that this threefold way is like an iron chain binding the feet of the man who tries to escape from the prison-house of this world. He who frees himself from it attains liberation.

∽ ∽ ∽

WHEN sandalwood is dipped in filthy water, its delicious fragrance may be overpowered by the smell of the filth. But as soon as you rub the sandalwood, the bad odor disappears and the air is filled with heavenly fragrance.

The heavenly fragrance of the Atman is overpowered by the foul odor of countless evil desires, which are like mud within us. Like sandalwood, its fragrance will fill the air when it has been cleansed by constant rubbing with the thought: "I am Brahman".

The sweet fragrance of the Atman is overpowered by innumerable cravings for the things of the senses. These cravings can be destroyed by devotion to the Atman; and then the light of the Atman becomes revealed.

As the mind gradually becomes devoted to the Atman, it frees itself by degrees from craving for sense-objects. When it has rid itself entirely of all craving, the vision of the Atman is no longer obstructed.

Through constant devotion to the Atman, the mind's impurities dissolve away. All cravings are obliterated. Strive, therefore, to destroy this illusion.

Tamas is overcome by both rajas and sattwa; rajas is overcome by sattwa; sattwa is overcome when the pure Atman shines. Therefore be established in sattwa and strive to destroy this illusion.

Be steadfast in your devotion, knowing that the body will certainly continue to live as long as it must. Strive with patience and perseverance to destroy this illusion.

Think: "I am Brahman; I am not the individual soul", and reject everything that is non-Atman. Strive thus to destroy this illusion which has been created in the past by your craving for sense-objects.

Learn the truth from the scriptures, reason upon it, and then know, by your own direct experience, that the Atman within you is the Atman in all. Strive thus to destroy this illusion, even to its last traces.

The wise man has not the least concern with getting and spending. Therefore strive to destroy this illusion, through constant and single-minded devotion to Brahman.

Meditate on the truth "That art Thou", and realize the identity of the Atman with Brahman. Strive to destroy this illusion and be established in the knowledge that Atman and Brahman are one.

With watchfulness and concentration you must strive to destroy this illusion, until all identification of the Atman with this body has completely ceased.

Even though you may have reached a stage at which the universe and its creatures appear as dream-images only, no longer seeming real, nevertheless, O prudent one, you must still strive ceaselessly to destroy this illusion.

Do not waste a moment in concern for worldly affairs or attraction to sense-objects. Remember Brahman even while you are asleep. Meditate upon the Atman within your own heart.

## False Identification

STOP identifying yourself with this corruptible physical body, born of the flesh of father and mother. Regard it as impure, as though it were an outcast. Attain the goal of life by realizing your unity with Brahman.

The air in a jar is one with the air everywhere. In like manner, your Atman is one with Brahman. O prudent one, lose all sense of separation and enter into silence.

Realize that you are one with the self-luminous Brahman, the ground of all existence. Reject the physical universe and the body, like pots of dirt.

The "I"-consciousness is now rooted in the body. Merge this consciousness in the Atman, which is absolute existence, knowledge and bliss. The consciousness of the subtle body is another limitation. Cast that off, also. Remain united with the Absolute forever.

The mirage of the universe is reflected in Brahman, like a city in a mirror. Know "I am that Brahman", and you will reach the goal of life.

The Atman is the reality. It is your true, primal self. It is pure consciousness, the one without a second, absolute bliss. It is beyond form and action. Realize your identity with it. Stop identifying yourself with the coverings of ignorance, which are like the masks assumed by an actor.

∽   ∽   ∽

THE universe of appearance is indeed unreal. The sense of ego must also be unreal, since we observe how it comes and goes. But we are conscious, also, of being the witness, the knower of everything. This consciousness does not belong to the ego-sense and the other perceptions which exist only for a moment at a time.

The Atman is the witness of the ego and the rest. It is present always, even in deep sleep. The scriptures also declare that the Atman is unborn and undying. It is, therefore, distinct from the gross and the subtle coverings.

The Atman must necessarily be changeless and eternal, since it is the knower of all that is changeable. The non-existence of the gross and subtle coverings can be experienced over and over again, when we dream or pass into deep sleep.

Cease, therefore, to identify yourself with this lump of flesh, the gross body, and with the ego, the subtle covering. Both of them are illusory. Know your Atman—the pure, infinite consciousness, eternally existent in the past, present and future. Thus you will find peace.

Cease to identify yourself with race, clan, name, form and walk of life. These belong to the body, the garment of decay. Abandon, also, the idea that you are the doer of actions or the thinker of thoughts. These belong to the ego, the subtle covering. Realize that you are that Being which is eternal happiness.

## The Ego

MAN'S life of bondage to the world of birth and death has many causes. The root of them all is the ego, the first-begotten child of ignorance.

As long as a man identifies himself with this wicked ego, there can be no possibility of liberation. For liberation is its very opposite.

Once freed from this eclipsing demon of an ego, man regains his true nature, just as the moon shines forth when freed from the darkness of an eclipse. He becomes pure, infinite, eternally blissful and self-luminous.

When a man's mind is overpowered by extreme ignorance, it creates the sense of ego by identifying itself with the coverings. When the ego is completely destroyed, the mind is cleared of the obstacles which obstruct its knowledge of oneness with Brahman.

The ego is a strong and deadly serpent, and the gunas are its three angry hoods. It lies coiled around the treasure of the bliss of Brahman, which it guards for its own use. The wise man, inspired by the holy scriptures, cuts off the three hoods with the sword of knowledge, and utterly destroys that serpent. Thus he enjoys the treasure of supreme bliss.

There is no hope of a man's recovery, as long as any trace of poison remains in his body. Similarly, the spiritual seeker cannot attain liberation as long as any trace of the ego remains within him.

Utterly destroy the ego. Control the many waves of distraction which it raises in the mind. Discern the reality and realize "I am That".

You are pure consciousness, the witness of all experiences. Your real nature is joy. Cease this very moment to identify yourself with the ego, the doer, which is created by ignornace. Its intelligence is only apparent, a reflection of the Atman, which is pure consciousness. It robs you of peace and joy in the Atman. By identifying yourself with it, you have fallen into the snare of the world—the miseries of birth, decay and death.

You are the Atman, the infinite Being, the pure, unchanging consciousness, which pervades everything. Your nature is bliss and your glory is without stain. Because you identify yourself with the ego, you are tied to birth and death. Your bondage has no other cause.

This ego is your enemy. It is like a thorn stuck in the throat of an eater. Destroy this enemy with the mighty sword of knowledge and be free to enjoy the sovereignty of your own empire, the bliss of the Atman.

Check all the activities of the ego, and the selfishness they involve. Attain the supreme reality, and be free from lust. Dwell in silence, and enjoy the bliss of the Atman. Lose all sense of separateness, and realize in Brahman your infinite nature.

This mighty ego may be cut down to the very roots. But if the mind feeds it, even for a moment, it will come to life again and cause a hundred mischiefs. It is like a storm-driven cloud in the rainy season.

Conquer this enemy, the ego. Give it no opportunity by letting your thoughts dwell upon sense-objects. Such thoughts give it life, as water gives life to a parched citron tree.

If you identify yourself with the body, lust will arise in you. Free yourself from consciousness of the body, and you will be freed from lust. Thus, if you are attached to this ego which keeps you separate from Brahman, you will run after pleasure in the objects of the senses. And this is the cause of bondage to birth and death.

## Cravings

THE more a man satisfies his cravings in the objective world, the more his cravings will increase. But if he controls them and ceases to gratify them, the seeds of craving will be destroyed. Therefore, let him gain self-control.

When craving grows stronger, self-control is lost. When self-control is lost, craving grows stronger than ever. A man who lives thus will never escape the wheel of birth and death.

Craving is intensified if we let our thoughts dwell upon sense-objects and seek temporary satisfaction in the objective world. In order to break the chain of recurring birth and death, the spiritual seeker must burn both these causes of craving to ashes.

Craving which is nourished in these two ways will bring bondage to the wheel of birth and death. But there is a way to destroy all three—this craving and both its causes. Under all circumstances, always, everywhere, and in all respects, you must look upon everything as Brahman, and Brahman alone. Strengthen your will to know the Reality, and these three will dissolve away.

Cease to find fulfillment of your cravings in the objective world, and you will stop dwelling on sense-objects. Stop dwelling on sense-objects, and your craving will be destroyed. When all craving has disappeared, that is liberation. It is called liberation-while-living.

∽ ∽ ∽

As THE thick darkness melts utterly away before the radiant glow of the rising sun, so the thirst for life in the ego is entirely removed when longing for knowledge of the Reality becomes intense.

When the lord of day ascends, darkness vanishes, with its net of evil. So, when the absolute bliss is experienced, there is no more bondage, nor any trace of sorrow.

Let this objective world vanish from your thoughts. Let your mind dwell in the Reality, which is full of joy. No matter whether you are regarding external appearances or meditating within yourself, be intently absorbed in Brahman. That is how you must pass your time, until the residue of your past karmas is worked out.

# Recollection

LET there be no negligence in your devotion to Brahman. Negligence in the practice of recollection is death—this has been declared by the seer, Sanatkumar, Brahma's son.

For a spiritual seeker, there is no greater evil than negligence in recollection. From it arises delusion. From delusion arises the sense of ego. From ego comes bondage, and from bondage misery.

A man may be learned, but if he is negligent in the practice of recollection he will turn toward the lures of the senses. The evil tendencies of his mind will seduce him, as a wicked woman seduces her lover.

When sedge is displaced on the surface of a pond, it closes in again at once. So Maya closes in even upon a wise man, if he ceases to practice recollection.

If the mind turns aside from Brahman, its ideal, and becomes ever so slightly caught in the sensuality of objects, it will continue to go downward, through negligence in recollection, like a ball dropped upon a flight of stairs.

If the mind is directed toward sense-objects, it dwells upon the pleasures which are derived from them. Indulgence in such thoughts excites craving. Because of craving, a man runs to gratify his desire.

Hence, to a man of spiritual discrimination, a knower of Brahman, there is no death but negligence in recollection. The man who is absorbed in recollection attains liberation. Therefore, make the greatest effort to remain absorbed in the Atman.

Through negligence in recollection, a man is distracted from awareness of his divine nature. He who is thus distracted falls—and the fallen always come to ruin. It is very hard for them to rise again.

## Rejection of Appearances

CEASE therefore to dwell upon sense-objects: that is the root of all evil. He who has won liberation in this life is liberated also when he gives up the body. The Yajur-Veda declares that a man is subject to fear as long as he sees the least difference between himself and Brahman.

Whenever a man—even if he has discrimination—sees the least distinction between himself and the infinite Brahman, fear will arise in him. Such difference is seen only because of ignorance.

Reason, sacred tradition, and hundreds of scriptural texts declare that the objective universe has no real existence. He who identifies himself with it encounters hosts upon hosts of sorrows.

He who is devoted to contemplation of the Reality becomes liberated and attains the eternal glory of the Atman. But he whose mind dwells upon the unreal, will lose himself.

The spiritual seeker must stop hunting after the unreal which causes bondage. He must stand firm in the vision of the Atman, remembering that "this Atman is myself". Steadfast devotion to Brahman and meditation upon one's identity with Brahman bring joy, and wipe out the immediate experience of suffering which is caused by ignorance.

The pursuit of sense-objects bears fruit in the increase of our evil tendencies, which grow worse and worse. We must know this by means of spiritual discrimination, and avoid thinking about sense-objects. Apply yourself constantly to meditation upon the Atman.

Refuse to dwell upon sense-objects, and peace will arise in your heart. When the heart is peaceful, the vision of the Atman comes. When the Atman has been directly realized, our bondage to this world is destroyed. Therefore, refusal to dwell upon sense-objects is the path to liberation.

If a man is learned, capable of discriminating between real and unreal, convinced of the authority of the scriptures, possessed of the vision of the Atman and desirous of liberation, how can he cling like a child to what is unreal and able to cause his downfall?

For him who is attached to the body and its pleasures, there can be no liberation. He who is liberated is free from attachment to the body and its pleasures. He who is asleep is not awake, and he who is awake is not asleep. These two states of consciousness are opposed to each other, by their very natures.

When a man knows the Atman, and sees it inwardly and outwardly as the ground of all things animate or inanimate, he has indeed reached liberation. He rejects all appearances as unreal and is established in the vision of the Atman, which is the Absolute, Infinite Being.

To see that one Atman as the ground of all appearances is the way to deliverance from bondage. There is no higher knowledge than to know that the Atman is one, and everywhere. A man realizes that the Atman is everywhere and in all things if he rejects appearances and devotes himself steadfastly to the Atman, the Eternal Being.

But how can a man reject appearances if he lives identified with the body, if his mind is attached to sense-objects, and if he pursues the fulfillment of his cravings? Only by strenuous effort can this rejection be accomplished. Practice spiritual discrimination, and be passionately devoted to the Atman. Renounce those selfish rewards which are obtained through the performance of actions and duties. Give up seeking pleasure in sense-objects. Desire nothing but possession of undying bliss.

In the scriptures, it is said: "When a man, who has heard the truth of Brahman from the lips of his teacher, becomes calm, self-controlled, satisfied, patient and deeply absorbed in contemplation, he realizes the Atman within his own heart and sees the Atman as all."

For such a seeker, the above passage prescribes deep contemplation of the Atman in order that the Atman in all things may be realized.

## The Rope and the Snake

IT IS impossible even for the wise to destroy the ego at a single blow—it is too firmly rooted in human nature; it continues, with its many cravings, through innumerable births. The ego is completely destroyed only in those who have become enlightened through attainment of the highest transcendental consciousness.

When a man's mind has become veiled in ignorance, the power of projection, whose nature is restlessness, causes him to identify himself with the ego. The ego seduces and distracts him with the desires which are its attributes.

It is hard to overcome the power of projection until the veiling power of ignorance is completely destroyed. When a man can distinguish as clearly between the Atman and external appearances as between milk and water, then the veil of ignorance which covers the Atman will vanish naturally. When the mind is no longer distracted by the mirage of sense-objects, every obstacle to realization of the Atman has undoubtedly been overcome.

When a man becomes illumined by knowledge, there arises within him perfect discrimination which clearly distinguishes the true Being, the Atman, from the external appearances. Thus he is freed from the bonds of delusion created by Maya and is no longer subject to death and rebirth in the world of change.

The knowledge that we are Brahman is like a fire which altogether consumes the thick forest of ignorance. When a man has realized his oneness with Brahman, how can he harbor any seed of death and rebirth?

When the vision of Reality comes, the veil of ignorance is completely removed. As long as we perceive things falsely, our false perception distracts us and makes us miserable. When our false perception is corrected, misery ends also.

For example, you see a rope and think it is a snake. As soon as you realize that the rope is a rope, your false perception of a snake ceases, and you are no longer distracted by the fear which it inspired. Therefore, the wise man who wishes to break his bondage must know the Reality.

Just as iron gives forth sparks when it is in contact with fire, so the mind appears to act and to perceive because of its contact with Brahman, which is consciousness itself. These powers of action and perception, which seem to belong to the mind, are unreal. They are as false as things seen in delusion, imagination and dream.

The modifications of Maya—ranging from the sense of ego down to the body and the sense-objects—are all unreal. They are unreal because they change from moment to moment. The Atman never changes.

The Atman is supreme, eternal, indivisible, pure consciousness, one without a second. It is the witness of the mind, intellect and other faculties. It is distinct from the gross and the subtle. It is the real I. It is the inner Being, the uttermost, everlasting joy.

Thus the wise man discriminates between the real and the unreal. His unsealed vision perceives the Real. He knows his own Atman to be pure indivisible consciousness. He is set free from ignorance, misery and the power of distraction. He enters directly into peace.

When the vision of the Atman, the one without a second, is attained through nirvikalpa samadhi, then the knots of the heart's ignorance are loosed completely and for ever.

"You", "I", "this"—such ideas of separateness originate in the impurity of the mind. But when the vision of the Atman—the supreme, the absolute, the one without a second—shines forth in samadhi, then all sense of separateness vanishes, because the Reality has been firmly apprehended.

## Samadhi

THE spiritual seeker who is possessed of tranquillity, self-control, mental poise and forbearance, devotes himself to the practice of contemplation, and meditates upon the Atman within himself as the Atman within all beings. Thus he completely destroys the sense of separateness which arises from the darkness of ignorance, and dwells in joy, identifying himself with Brahman, free from distracting thoughts and selfish occupations.

Those who echo borrowed teachings are not free from the world. But those who have attained samadhi by merging the external universe, the sense-organs, the mind and the ego in the pure consciousness of the Atman—they alone are free from the world, with its bonds and snares.

The one Atman appears as many, because of the variety of its outer coverings. When these unreal coverings dissolve away, the Atman alone exists. Let the wise man therefore devote himself to the attainment of nirvikalpa samadhi, in order that the coverings may melt out of his consciousness.

If a man loves Brahman with an exclusive and steadfast devotion, he becomes Brahman. By thinking of nothing but the wasp, the cockroach is changed into a wasp.

Just as the cockroach turns into a wasp because

it gives up every other activity and thinks of nothing but that insect, so the spiritual seeker who meditates on the reality of the Atman becomes the Atman, because of his steadfast devotion.

The true nature of the Atman is extremely subtle. It cannot be perceived by the gross mind. It must be known in the state of samadhi which can be attained only by those noble souls whose minds are purified and who possess an extraordinary power of spiritual discrimination.

As gold which has been refined in hot fire is purged of dross and restored to its own nature, so, through meditation, the mind purges itself of the dross of sattwa, rajas and tamas, and attains Brahman.

When the mind, thus purged by ceaseless meditation, is merged in Brahman, the state of samadhi is attained. In that state there is no sense of duality. The undivided joy of Brahman is experienced.

When a man reaches samadhi, all the knots of his desires are cut through and he is freed from the law of karma. Brahman is revealed to him, internally and externally, everywhere and always, without any further effort on his part.

It is a hundred times better to reflect on the truth of Brahman than merely to hear about it from the scriptures. And meditation is a hundred thousand times better than reflection. But nirvikalpa samadhi is infinitely the best of all.

In nirvikalpa samadhi—and in no other state— the true nature of Brahman is clearly and definitely revealed. In any other state, the mind remains unstable: it is filled with distracting thoughts.

Therefore remain constantly absorbed in the consciousness of the Atman within you. Control your senses and let your mind be tranquil. Gain the clear vision of your oneness with Brahman and thereby destroy the ignorance which Maya has created from time without beginning.

## Inner and Outer Control

THESE are the first steps toward union with Brahman—control of speech, refusal to accept unnecessary gifts, abandonment of worldly ambitions and desires, continuous devotion to Brahman.

Be devoted to Brahman and you will be able to control your senses. Control your senses and you will gain mastery over your mind. Master your mind, and the sense of ego will be dissolved. In this manner, the yogi achieves an unbroken realization of the joy of Brahman. Therefore let the seeker strive to give his heart to Brahman.

Control speech by mental effort; control the mind by the faculty of discrimination; control this faculty by the individual will; merge individuality in the infinite absolute Atman and reach supreme peace.

The body, the vital energy, the sense-organs, the mind, the intellect and the ego—these are the coverings of the Atman. When a man is identified with any one of these coverings, he assumes its nature and aspect.

When this identification ceases, the meditative man easily detaches himself from these coverings and experiences perpetually the fullness of ever-lasting joy.

To detach ourselves completely from all these coverings is to possess both inner and outer renunciation. This renunciation can only be practiced by one who is endowed with dispassion. The dispassionate man who longs for liberation can practice both inner and outer renunciation.

External attachment is attachment to sense-objects. Internal attachment is self-identification with the ego and the modifications of the mind. The dispassionate man, absorbingly devoted to Brahman, is alone able to renounce both.

Know, O wise one, that a man needs dispassion and discrimination as a bird needs its two wings. Without them, a man cannot reach the top of the vine from which flows the nectar of liberation. He can never get to it by any other means.

Only the man who has intense dispassion can attain samadhi. He who has attained samadhi lives in a state of constant illumination. The illumined heart is liberated from bondage. The liberated man alone experiences eternal joy.

For the man of self-mastery, dispassion is the only source of happiness. If this is combined with the awakening of the pure knowledge of the Atman, a man becomes independent of all else. This is the door to the enjoyment of that ever-youthful maiden who is called liberation. If, therefore, you seek the highest good, practice inner and outer dispassion and maintain a constant awareness of the eternal Atman.

Shun the craving for sensual life like poison, for it is death. Give up pride of caste, family and rank and abstain from deeds of self-interest. Give up the delusion that you are the body or any of the coverings—they are all unreal. Keep your mind recollected in the Atman. In truth, you are Brahman, the witness unfettered by the mind, the one without a second, the highest.

Fasten the mind upon Brahman, your goal. Do not allow the sense-organs to function externally; compel them to remain in their respective centers. Keep the body straight and firm. Take no thought for its maintenance. Be utterly devoted to Brahman, and realize that yourself and Brahman are one. Drink the joy of Brahman unceasingly. The springs of that joy never run dry. What use is there in the things of this world? They are empty of happiness.

Do not let your mind dwell on any thought which is not of the Atman. To do so is evil, a cause of misery. Meditate on the Atman, whose nature is bliss. That is the way to liberation.

The self-luminous Atman, the witness of all, is ever-present within your own heart. This Atman stands apart from all that is unreal. Know it to be yourself, and meditate upon it unceasingly.

Let there be an uninterrupted communion with the Atman, free from all distracting thoughts. In this way you will realize, without a doubt, that the Atman is your real nature.

Hold fast to the truth that you are the Atman. Give up identifying yourself with the ego, or any of the coverings. Remain completely indifferent to them, as though they were broken jars of clay.

Fix the purified mind upon the Atman, the

witness, the pure consciousness. Strive gradually to calm your mind. Then you will attain the vision of the infinite Atman.

## The One

MEDITATE upon the Atman as indivisible, infinite, like the all-pervading ether. Know it to be separate from the body, the senses, the vital energy, the mind and the ego—those limitations imposed upon us by our ignorance.

The ether—though it fills hundreds of vessels, such as jars and pots of grain and rice, and seems various and divided—is really one, not many. So also the pure Atman, when it is freed from the limitations of ego and mind, is one and one only.

All things—from Brahma[1] the creator down to a single blade of grass—are the apparently diverse names and forms of the one Atman. They are simply appearances, and not real. Therefore meditate upon the Atman as one and infinite.

The Atman is the ground and the reality. This appearance of a universe is only seen through our deluded eyes. When true knowledge arises, the Atman is revealed as existence itself, and the apparent universe cannot be seen apart from it. You may mistake a rope for a snake, if you are deluded. But, when the delusion passes, you realize that the imagined snake was none other than the rope. So also this universe is none other than the Atman.

[1]Brahma, one of the Hindu trinity, the creator, as distinct from Brahman, God in his impersonal, absolute aspect.

I, THE Atman, am Brahma. I am Visnu. I am Shiva.[2] I am this universe. Nothing is, but I am.

I dwell within; I am without. I am before and behind. I am in the south and I am in the north. I am above and I am below.

The wave, the foam, the eddy and the bubble are all essentially water. Similarly, the body and the ego are really nothing but pure consciousness. Everything is essentially consciousness, purity and joy.

This entire universe of which we speak and think is nothing but Brahman. Brahman dwells beyond the range of Maya. There is nothing else. Are jars, pots and vessels distinct from the clay of which they are made? Man drinks the wine of Maya, becomes deluded and begins to see things as separate from each other, so that he talks of "you" and "I".

The scripture says: "The Infinite is where one sees nothing else, hears nothing else, knows nothing else." In the Infinite, the scripture tells us, there is no duality—thereby correcting our false idea that existence is manifold.

I am Brahman, the supreme, all-pervading like the ether, stainless, indivisible, unbounded, unmoved, unchanging. I have neither inside nor outside. I alone am. I am one without a second. What else is there to be known?

What more remains to be said? I am none other than Brahman. Brahman is this universe and all things that exist within it. The scriptures declare that there is nothing else but Brahman. Those

[2]The Hindu trinity: Brahma, the creator; Vishnu, the preserver; Shiva, the destroyer.

who are illumined by the knowledge "I am Brahman" renounce their attachment to this apparent universe. It is certain indeed that these illumined ones live in constant union with Brahman, the pure blissful consciousness.

## Deliverance

RENOUNCE all earthly hopes and physical pleasures by ceasing to identify yourself with the gross body. Next, you must cease also to identify yourself with the subtle body. Realize that you are Brahman, whose form is bliss eternal, whose glories the scriptures declare. Thus you may live in union with Brahman.

As long as a man loves this mortal body, he remains impure, he is troubled by his enemies in all manner of ways, he is still subject to rebirth, disease and death. But if he will meditate upon the Atman as pure, unchangeable, the essence of goodness, he will be delivered from all evil. The scriptures also confirm this truth.

Cease to identify yourself mistakenly with all those coverings, such as the ego, etc., which overlie the Atman. Brahman alone remains— supreme, infinite, changeless, the one without a second.

## The Phantom World

WHEN the mind is completely absorbed in the supreme Being—the Atman, the Brahman, the Absolute—then the world of appearances vanishes. Its existence is no more than an empty word.

The world of appearances is a mere phantom; there is but one Reality. It is changeless, formless and absolute. How can it be divided?

There is neither seer nor seeing nor seen. There is but one Reality—changeless, formless and absolute. How can it be divided?

There is but one Reality—like a brimming ocean in which all appearances are dissolved. It is changeless, formless and absolute. How can it be divided?

Into it, the causes of our delusion melt away, as darkness melts into light. It is supreme, absolute, one without a second. How can it be divided?

There is but one supreme Reality. It is the very self of unity. It cannot possibly be divided into many. If multiplicity is real, and not merely apparent, why does no one ever experience it while enjoying dreamless sleep?

The universe no longer exists after we have awakened into the highest consciousness in the eternal Atman, which is Brahman, devoid of any distinction or division. At no time—either past, present or future—is there really a snake within the rope or a drop of water in the mirage.

The scriptures declare that this relative universe is only an appearance. The Absolute is non-dual. In dreamless sleep, also, the universe disappears.

It is our delusion which superimposes the universe upon Brahman. But the wise know that this universe has no separate reality. It is identical with Brahman, its ground. The rope may appear to be a snake, but the apparent difference between rope and snake only lasts as long as delusion persists.

This delusion of difference has its origin in the gross mind. When the mind is transcended, it ceases. Therefore let your mind be absorbed in contemplation of the Atman, the reality, your inmost essence.

## Union with Brahman

WHEN the mind achieves perfect union with Brahman, the wise man realizes Brahman entirely within his own heart. Brahman is beyond speech or thought. It is the pure, eternal consciousness. It is absolute bliss. It is incomparable and immeasurable. It is ever-free, beyond all action, boundless as the sky, indivisible and absolute.

When the mind achieves perfect union with Brahman, the wise man realizes Brahman entirely within his own heart. Brahman is beyond cause and effect. It is the reality beyond all thought. It is eternally the same, peerless, outside the range of any mental conception. It is revealed by the sacred scriptures and it is forever revealing itself in us through our sense of ego.

When the mind achieves perfect union with Brahman, the wise man realizes Brahman entirely within his own heart. Brahman knows no decay or death. It is the Reality without beginning and without end. It is like a vast sheet of water, shoreless and calm. It is beyond the play of the gunas. It is one, the eternal, forever tranquil.

Be absorbed in union with your true Being, and behold the Atman of infinite glory. Escape the bondage and the rotten stench of worldliness. Make a strenuous effort and attain liberation.

Then you will not have been born into this world
in vain.

Meditate upon the Atman, your true Being,
which is free from all coverings and limitations,
the infinite existence, knowledge and bliss, the
one without a second. Thus you will escape from
the wheel of birth and death.

## Detachment

THE effects of past actions cause the illumined
seer to continue to live on in the body—but to
him the body is only an appearance, like a man's
shadow. And when he puts off the body as a
corpse he will never again be born into another
body.

Realize the Atman, the eternal pure consciousness and bliss. Detach yourself completely from
this covering, the body, which is sluggish and
foul. Having done this, never think of it again. To
remember one's own vomit is merely disgusting.

The truly wise man burns his ignorance with all
its effects in the fire of Brahman—the Absolute,
the Eternal, the very Self. He then remains established in the knowledge of the Atman, the eternal
pure consciousness and bliss.

A cow is indifferent to the garland which is
hung around her neck. The knower of Brahman is
indifferent to the fate of this body, which continues to live on through the effect of his past
actions. His mind is absorbed in the blissful
Brahman.

The knower of Brahman has realized his true

Being, the Atman, which is endless joy. What motive or desire can he possibly have to attach himself any longer to this body and to nourish it?

To taste, within his own heart and in the external world, the endless bliss of the Atman—such is the reward obtained by the yogi who has reached perfection and liberation in this life.

## Dispassion

THE fruit of dispassion is illumination; the fruit of illumination is the stilling of desire; the fruit of stilled desire is experience of the bliss of the Atman, whence follows peace.

The first steps are worthless unless the path be followed to the end. Dispassion, supreme satisfaction and incomparable bliss must follow one another naturally.

It is well known that the fruit of illumination is the cessation of suffering. A man may do many evil deeds through ignorance. But how can he continue to do evil when discrimination has been awakened within him?

Illumination causes a man to turn away from the evil and the unreal; attachment to these is the result of ignorance. Compare a man who knows what a mirage is with a man who is ignorant of its nature. The former turns away from it; the latter runs toward it to satisfy his thirst. The man of realization is no longer lured by the world of appearances—that is his evident reward.

When the heart's knot of ignorance is cut right through, a man is freed from all craving for material objects. When this has happened, is there anything in the world which can possibly cause him to feel any attachment?

When the objects of enjoyment fail to arouse any craving, that is perfect renunciation. When there is no longer any sense of ego, that is perfect knowledge. When the mind is absorbed in Brahman and no longer distracted by any other thought, that is perfect self-withdrawal.

A man who remains continually absorbed in the consciousness of Brahman is freed from the tyranny of the objective world. The enjoyments which others find so irresistible he values as little as a small baby would, or a man who was sound asleep. When, at moments, he becomes conscious of this world, he looks upon it as a world of dreams. He enjoys the fruits of endless merit. Such a man is blessed indeed. He is esteemed on earth.

The self-controlled man is said to be illumined when he enjoys eternal bliss. He is entirely merged in Brahman. He knows himself to be the unchangeable Reality, which is beyond action.

## Illumination

THE state of illumination is described as follows: There is a continuous consciousness of the unity of Atman and Brahman. There is no longer any identification of the Atman with its coverings. All sense of duality is obliterated. There is pure, unified consciousness. The man who is well established in this consciousness is said to be illumined.

A man is said to be free even in this life when be is established in illumination. His bliss is unending. He almost forgets this world of appearances.

Even though his mind is dissolved in Brahman, he is fully awake, free from the ignorance of waking life. He is fully conscious, but free from any craving. Such a man is said to be free even in this life.

For him, the sorrows of this world are over. Though he possesses a finite body, he remains united with the Infinite. His heart knows no anxiety. Such a man is said to be free even in this life.

Though he lives in the body, it seems merely like a shadow following him. He is no longer troubled by the thought of "I" and "mine". Such are the characteristics of a man who is free even in this life.

He does not care to delve into the past. He is not interested in scanning the future. He is indifferent to the present. That is how you may know the man who is free even in this life.

Good and evil appear to exist in the world. Persons and objects seem to be distinct from each other. Nevertheless, he regards everything from the standpoint of equality, for he sees Brahman in all. That is how you may know the man who is free even in this life.

Good or evil fortune may come. He regards them both with indifference, and remains unaffected by either. That is how you may know the man who is free even in this life.

Because his mind is continually engaged in tasting the bliss of Brahman, he is unable to distinguish between the internal and the external. That is how you may know the man who is free even in this life.

Life flows by: he watches it like a disinterested spectator. He does not identify himself with the body, sense-organs, etc. He has risen above the idea of duty. That is how you may know the man who is free even in this life.

By the help of the living words of the scriptures, he has realized his oneness with Brahman. He is no longer bound to rebirth. That is how you may know the man who is free even in this life.

He never identifies himself with the body or the sense-organs. He has no feeling of ownership. That is how you may know the man who is free even in this life.

Through his transcendental vision he has realized that there is no difference between man and Brahman, or between Brahman and the universe—for he sees that Brahman is all. That is how you may know the man who is free even in this life.

Holy men may honor him, evil men may insult him—his feelings are the same. That is how you may know the man who is free even in this life.

Rivers flow into the ocean, but the ocean is not disturbed. Sense-objects flow into his mind, but he feels no reaction, for he lives in the consciousness of the one Reality. He is free indeed, even in this life.

## Breaking the Dream

HE WHO has known the reality of Brahman cannot continue to feel attachment to this word. He who feels attachment has not known Brahman. He remains deluded and sensebound.

Of a man who has known Brahman it cannot be said that he is still attached to sense-objects because of the strong impressions and old habits of his past desires. No—his desires and tendencies are wiped out, because he has realized his identity with Brahman.

Even a very lustful man feels no desire when he is in the presence of his mother. In the same manner a man is freed from worldliness if he has realized Brahman, the infinite bliss.

The scriptures declare that even the man of meditation is conscious of the external world, because of tendencies created by his former way of life. These tendencies are said to be working themselves out in him.

As long as a man experiences pleasure and pain, his past tendencies will persist. Every effect is preceded by a cause. Where there is no cause, there is no effect.

When a man wakes from his dream, his dream-actions vanish into nothingness. When a man wakes to the knowledge that he is Brahman, all accumulated causes, all past actions performed in the course of millions and millions of lives, are dissolved away.

While a man is asleep, he may dream that he is doing good deeds or committing dreadful sins. But, when the dream breaks, how can these dream-actions lead him either to heaven or to hell?

The Atman is forever free and pure and untouchable as the ether. He who has realized the

Atman can never be bound by his actions, past, present or to come.

The ether enclosed within a jar is not affected by the smell of the wine. The Atman within its coverings is not affected by the properties of the coverings.

## The Arrow will not stop

*The Disciple:*

I understand that after the attainment of illumination no action can affect the Atman. But what about actions done before the dawn of knowledge? Knowledge cannot cancel their effects. An arrow shot at a mark cannot be turned aside.

Suppose you mistake a cow for a tiger and shoot at it. The arrow will not stop when you discover that the cow is not a tiger. It will strike the cow.

*The Master:*

Yes, you are right. Past actions are very powerful if they have already begun to produce their effects. They must exhaust their power through actual experience, even in the case of an illumined soul. The fire of knowledge destroys the whole accumulation of present and future karmas and of past karmas which have not yet begun to produce effects. But it cannot destroy those past karmas which have already begun to produce effects. However, none of these karmas can really affect those who have realized their identity with Brahman and live continually absorbed in that consciousness. Such men have become united with Brahman, the one beyond all attributes.

The seer lives absorbed in the consciousness of the Atman. He has realized his identity with Brahman. Brahman is pure and free from the qualities which belong to the gross and subtle coverings. Past karmas belong to these coverings—therefore they do not affect the seer. When a man is awake, he is no longer in bondage to the apparent world of his dreams.

The man who has awakened no longer identifies himself with his dream-body, his dream-actions, or the objects of his dream. He comes to himself simply by waking up.

He does not try to maintain that the objects of his dream are real, nor does he seek to possess them. If he still pursues the objects of the dream-world, then he has certainly not yet awakened from his sleep.

Similarly, he who has awakened to the knowledge of Brahman lives absorbed in union with the eternal Atman. He sees nothing else. True, he has to eat, he has to sustain his body as long as he lives in the world. But such actions are performed, as it were, from memory. They are like the remembered actions of a dream.

Birth into a body is the result of karma. It may be said, therefore, that past actions only affect the body. The Atman is beginningless. It cannot be said to be born as a result of karma. And so it is unreasonable to think that karma can affect the Atman.

The infallible words of the scriptures declare that "the Atman is unborn, eternal, never subject to decay." How, therefore, can any karma be supposed to affect the man who lives in the consciousness of the Atman?

The accumulated causes due to past actions affect a man who identifies himself with the body. The illumined soul knows that this identification is false. That is why he is not affected by such karma.

It is foolish, even, to think that the accumulated causes due to past actions can affect the body. How can this body be real when it has only an illusory existence? How can something unreal have a birth? How can something die which has never been born? How can actions or their effects affect what is unreal?

When knowledge drawns, ignorance and the effects of ignorance vanish. The ignorant man may ask, "If that is so, how can the body of an illumined soul continue to exist?" But when the scriptures say that the continuance of the body is caused by past actions they are simply explaining things in a way which the ignorant can understand. They do not mean to prove the reality of the body and the other coverings from the standpoint of an illumined soul.

## Brahman is All

FROM the standpoint of the illumined soul, Brahman fills everything—beginningless, endless, immeasurable, unchanging, one without a second. In Brahman there is no diversity whatsoever.

Brahman is pure existence, pure consciousness, eternal bliss, beyond action, one without a second. In Brahman there is no diversity whatsoever.

Brahman is the innermost consciousness, filled full of endless bliss, infinite, omnipresent, one without a second. In Brahman there is no diversity whatsoever.

Brahman cannot be avoided, since it is everywhere. Brahman cannot be grasped, since it is transcendent. It cannot be contained, since it contains all things. It is one without a second. In Brahman there is no diversity whatsoever.

Brahman is without parts or attributes. It is subtle, absolute, taintless, one without a second. In Brahman there is no diversity whatsoever.

Brahman is indefinable, beyond the range of mind and speech, one without a second. In Brahman there is no diversity whatsoever.

Brahman is reality itself; established in its own glory; pure, absolute consciousness, having no equal, one without a second. In Brahman there is no diversity whatsoever.

ᦠ   ᦠ   ᦠ

THE spiritual seekers, those great-hearted souls who have freed themselves from all cravings, casting aside sensual pleasures, tranquil and self-controlled—they realize this supreme truth of Brahman. They attain union with Brahman and reach the highest bliss.

You, too, must discriminate and realize the supreme truth of Brahman. Realize the true nature of the Atman as the sum of all bliss. Shake off the delusions which you own mind has created. Thus you will become free and illumined. You will make your life blessed.

Calm your mind utterly and attain samadhi. Then you will have open vision, seeing clearly the truth of the Atman. From the lips of your teacher you have learned of the truth of Brahman as it is revealed in the scriptures. Now you must realize that truth directly and immediately. Then only will your heart be free from any doubt.

ശ    ശ    ശ

How are you to know for certain that you are liberated from the bondage of ignorance and have realized the Atman, which is absolute existence, pure consciousness and abiding bliss? The words of the scriptures, your own power of reasoning and the teaching of your master should all help to convince you—but the only absolute proof is direct and immediate experience, within your own soul.

Bondage and liberation, satisfaction and anxiety, sickness and renewed health, hunger and so forth—these are matters of personal experience. You know yourself. Others can only guess at your condition.

Teachers and scriptures can stimulate spirtual awareness. But the wise disciple crosses the ocean of his ignorance by direct illumination, through the grace of God.

Gain experience directly. Realize God for yourself. Know the Atman as the one indivisible Being, and become perfect. Free you mind from all distractions and dwell in the consciousness of the Atman.

This is the final declaration of Vedanta: Brahman is all—this universe and every creature.

To be liberated is to live in Brahman, the undivided reality. Brahman is one without a second, as the scriptures bear witness.

## The Disciple Rejoices

THE disciple listened attentively to the words of his teacher. He learned the supreme truth of Brahman, to which the scriptures bear witness, and confirmed it by the aid of his own reasoning powers. He then withdrew his senses from the objective world and concentrated his mind upon the Atman. His body appeared as immovable as a rock.

His mind was completely absorbed in Brahman. After a while, he returned to normal consciousness. Then, out of the fullness of his joy, he spoke:

The ego has disappeared. I have realized my identity with Brahman and so all my desires have melted away. I have risen above my ignorance and my knowledge of this seeming universe. What is this joy that I feel? Who shall measure it? I know nothing but joy, limitless, unbounded!

The ocean of Brahman is full of nectar—the joy of the Atman. The treasure I have found there cannot be described in words. The mind cannot conceive of it. My mind fell like a hailstone into that vast expanse of Brahman's ocean. Touching one drop of it, I melted away and became one with Brahman. And now, though I return to human consciousness, I abide in the joy of the Atman.

Where is this universe? Who took it away? Has it merged into something else? A while ago, I beheld it—now it exists no longer. This is wonderful indeed!

Here is the ocean of Brahman, full of endless joy. How can I accept or reject anything? Is there anything apart or distinct from Brahman?

Now, finally and clearly, I know that I am the Atman, whose nature is eternal joy. I see nothing, I hear nothing, I know nothing that is separate from me.

ᔆ ᔆ ᔆ

I BOW down to you, O great soul, my master! You are free from all attachment, the greatest of the wise and the good. You are the embodiment of eternal bliss. Your compssion is infinite, a sea without a shore.

Your eyes are full of mercy. Their glance is like a flood of moonbeams, refreshing the weariness of my mortality, the pain of my bondage to human birth and death. In one instant, by your grace, I have found this inexhaustible, undivided treasure—the Atman, the ever-blissful.

I am blessed indeed! I have achieved life's only purpose. The dragon of rebirth can never seize me now. The Infinite is mine. I recognize my true nature in eternal joy. And all this through your mercy!

ᔆ ᔆ ᔆ

NOTHING binds me to this world. I no longer identify myself with the physical body or the mind. I am one with the Atman, the undying. I am the Atman—infinite, pure, eternal, at peace forever.

I am neither he who acts nor he who experiences the results of action. I am beyond action and am changeless. My nature is pure consciousness. I am absolute reality, eternal goodness.

It is not I who see, hear, speak, act, suffer or enjoy. I am the Atman, eternal, ever-living, beyond action, unbounded, unattached—nothing but pure, infinite consciousness.

I am neither this object, nor that. I am That which makes all objects manifest. I am supreme, eternally pure. I am neither inward nor outward. I am the infinte Brahman, one without a second.

I am Reality, without beginning, without equal. I have no part in the illusion of "I" and "You", "this" and "that". I am Brahman, one without a second, bliss without end, the eternal, unchanging Truth.

I am the Lord and refuge of all. I am the destroyer of all sins and impurities. I am pure, indivisible consciousness. I am the witness of all things. I have no other lord but myself. I am free from the sense of "I" and "mine".

I dwell within all beings as the Atman, the pure consciousness, the ground of all phenomena, internal and external. I am both the enjoyer and that which is enjoyed. In the days of my ignorance, I used to think of these as being separate from myself. Now I know that I am All.

In myself is the ocean of joy, infinite, undivided. The wind of Maya plays over it, creating and dissolving the appearances of this world, like waves.

Mistaking the appearance for the reality, people ignorantly imagine that I am enclosed within a bodily and a mental form. In the same way, they imagine Time, which is indivisible and continuous, to be divided into cycles, years and seasons.

But no matter what the imagination of deluded and ignorant fools may superimpose upon the Reality, the Reality remains untainted. The mighty river of water in the mirage cannot wet the dry desert.

Like the ether, I cannot be tainted. Like the sun, I am other than the objects I reveal. Like the mountain, I stand immovable. Like the ocean, I am boundless.

The sky is not confined by its clouds. I am not confined by the body. How, therefore, can I be affected by the states of waking, dreaming or dreamless sleep? They are merely bodily conditions.

My outward form comes and goes. It acts and tastes the fruits of its actions. It withers and it dies. But I remain, like a great mountain, firm and immovable forever.

I know neither desire nor the ending of desire—for I am the same always, incapable of division. How can any action be possible for the one who is eternal, universal, complete and infinite as the sky? What should he strive for?

I am without organs, without form, without mind. I am untouched by change. I am the undivided, blissful consciousness. How can I become involved in action, either righteous or sinful?

Therefore, the scriptures declare that "the Atman remains equally untouched by good and by evil".

A man is other than his shadow. No matter what touches his shadow—hot or cold, good or bad—he remains completely untouched.

The properties of the objects observed do not affect the witness who stands apart from them, without attachment. In the same manner, the properties of a room do not affect the lamp which reveals them.

The sun witnesses actions, but is distinct from them. The fire burns all things, but is distinct from them. The rope is mistaken for a snake, but remains a rope. So also I—the unchanging Atman, the pure consciousness—am distinct from this seeming form.

I neither act nor make others act, I neither experience nor make other experience, I neither see nor make others see. I am the Atman, self-luminous, transcendent.

The sun is reflected upon water. Water moves, and the fool thinks that the sun is moving. The Atman is reflected upon the physical and mental bodies. The bodies move and act, and the fool thinks: "I act, I experience, I am killed".

This body may drop dead in water or on land. I am not affected by that. The ether in a jar is not affected when the jar is broken.

To act or to enjoy, to be dull-witted or cunning or intoxicated, to be free or in bondage—all these are transient conditions of the intellect. They have nothing to do with the Atman, which is Brahman, the absolute, the one without a second. Let the Maya undergo ten, a hundred, a thousand transformations—what do they matter to me, who have no part in them? Can a cloud stain the sky?

This whole universe—from Maya down to the outward physical forms—is seen as a mere shadow of Brahman. I am that Brahman, one without a second, subtle as ether, without beginning or end.

I am that Brahman, one without a second, the ground of all existences. I make all things manifest. I give form to all things. I am within all things, yet nothing can taint me. I am eternal, pure, unchangeable, absolute.

I am that Brahman, one without a second. Maya, the many-seeming, is merged in me. I am beyond the grasp of thought, the essence of all things. I am the truth. I am knowledge. I am infinite. I am absolute bliss.

I am beyond action, the reality which cannot change. I have neither part nor form. I am absolute. I am eternal. Nothing sustains me, I stand alone. I am one without a second.

I am the soul of the universe. I am all things, and above all things. I am one without a second. I am pure consciousness, single and universal. I am joy. I am life everlasting.

Ever and ever again, I salute you, most noble lord, my master. By the supreme majesty of your grace, I have found this blessed state. I am ruler of the kingdom of myself.

∾　∾　∾

UNTIL now, I have been dreaming. In my dream, I wandered through the forest of illusion, from birth to birth, beset by all kinds of troubles and miseries, subject to reincarnation, decay and death. The tiger of ego attacked me cruelly, without ceasing. Now, by your infinite compassion, O master, you have wakened me from my dream. You have set me free forever.

Salutations to you, O great master. You are one with Brahman. You are one with the shining Light that casts this shadow of a world.

## The Crest Jewel

THE worthy disciple has found the joy of the Atman in samadhi and awakened forever to consciousness of Reality. Now he prostrates himself before his great master. The master, glad at heart, speaks to him again, in the following memorable words:

Our perception of the universe is a continuous perception of Brahman, though the ignorant man is not aware of this. Indeed, this universe is nothing but Brahman. See Brahman everywhere, under all circumstances, with the eye of the spirit and a tranquil heart. How can the physical eyes see anything but physical objects? How can the mind of the enlightened man think of anything other than the Reality?

How could a wise man reject the experience of supreme bliss and take delight in mere outward forms? When the moon shines in its exceeding beauty, who would care to look at a painted moon?

Experience of the unreal offers us no satisfaction, nor any escape from misery. Find satisfaction, therefore, in the experience of the sweet bliss of Brahman. Devote yourself to the Atman and live happily forever.

O noble soul, this is how you must pass your days—see the Atman everywhere, enjoy the bliss of the Atman, fix your thought upon the Atman, the one without a second.

The Atman is one, absolute, indivisible. It is pure consciousness. To imagine many forms within it is like imagining palaces in the air. Therefore, know that you are the Atman, ever-blissful, one without a second, and find the ultimate peace. Remain absorbed in the joy which is silence.

This state of silence is a state of entire peace, in which the intellect ceases to occupy itself with the unreal. In this silence, the great soul who knows and is one with Brahman enjoys unmingled bliss forever.

To the man who has realized the Atman as his true being and who has tasted the innermost bliss of the Atman, there is no more excellent joy than this state of silence, in which all cravings are dumb.

No matter what he is doing—walking, standing, sitting or lying down—the illumined seer whose delight is the Atman lives in joy and freedom.

When a great soul has found perfect tranquillity be freeing his mind from all distracting thoughts and completely realizing Brahman, then he no longer needs sacred places, moral disciplines, set hours, postures, directions or objects for his meditation. His knowledge of the Atman depends upon no special circumstances or conditions.

In order to know that a jar is a jar are any special conditions required? Only that our means of perception, the eyes, shall be free from defect. This alone revels the object.

The Atman is eternally present. It is revealed by transcendental experience, which is not dependent upon place, time or rituals of self-purification.

I do not require any special condition or proof in order to know that my name is Devadatta. Similarly, for a knower of Brahman, the knowledge that "I am Brahman" does not require any proof.

The Atman, shining with its own light, causes this apparent universe. But how can anything in this universe reveal the Atman? Apart from the Atman, these appearances are worthless, bodiless, unreal.

The Vedas, the Puranas, all scriptures and all living creatures only exist because the Atman exists. How then can any of them reveal the Atman, which is the revealer of everything?

 ✍ ✍ ✍

THIS Atman shines with its own light. Its power is infinite. It is beyond sense-knowledge. It is the source of all experience. He who knows the Atman is free from every kind of bondage. He is full of glory. He is the greatest of the great.

The things perceived by the senses cause him neither grief nor pleasure. He is not attached to them. Neither does he shun them. Constantly delighting in the Atman he is always at play within himself. He tastes the sweet, unending bliss of the Atman and is satisfied.

The child plays with his toys, forgetting even hunger and physical pain. In like manner, the knower of Brahman takes his delight in the Atman, fogetting all thought of "I" and "mine".

He gets his food easily by begging alms, without anxiety or care. He drinks from the clear stream. He lives unfettered and independent. He sleeps without fear in the forest or on the cremation-ground. He does not need to wash or dry his clothes, for he wears none. The earth is his bed. He walks the highway of Vedanta. His playmate is Brahman, the everlasting.

The knower of the Atman does not identify himself with his body. He rests within it, as if within a carriage. If people provide him with comforts and luxuries, he enjoys them and plays with them like a child. He bears no outward mark of a holy man. He remains quite unattached to the things of this world.

He may wear costly clothing, or none. He may be dressed in deer or tiger skin or clothed in pure knowledge. He may seem like a madman, or like a child, or sometimes like an unclean spirit. Thus, he wanders the earth.

The man of contemplation walks alone. He lives desireless amidst the objects of desire. The Atman is his eternal satisfaction. He sees the Atman present in all things.

Sometimes he appears to be a fool, sometimes a wise man. Sometimes he seems splendid as a king, sometimes feeble-minded. Sometimes he is calm and silent. Sometimes he draws men to him, as a python attracts its prey. Sometimes people honor him greatly, sometimes they insult him. Sometimes they ignore him. That is how the illumined soul lives, always absorbed in the highest bliss.

He has no riches, yet he is always contented. He is helpless, yet of mighty power. He enjoys nothing, yet he is continually rejoicing. He has no equal, yet he sees all men as his equals.

He acts, yet is not bound by his action. He reaps the fruit of past actions, yet is unaffected by them. He has a body, but does not identify himself with it. He appears to be an individual, yet he is present in all things, everywhere.

The knower of Brahman, who lives in freedom from body-consciousness, is never touched by pleasure or pain, good or evil.

If a man identifies himself with the gross and subtle coverings within which he dwells, he will experience pleasure and pain, good or evil. But nothing is either good or evil to the contemplative sage, because he has realized the Atman and his bonds have fallen from him.

During a solar eclipse, the sun is hidden by the moon. The ignorant, who do not understand what has happened, say that the sun has been swallowed up by a demon—but the sun can never be swallowed up.

In the same manner, the ignorant see the body of a knower of Brahman and identify him with it. Actually, he is free from the body and every other kind of bondage. To him, the body is merely a shadow.

He dwells in the body, but regards it as a thing apart from himself—like the cast-off skin of a snake. The body moves hither and thither, impelled by the vital force.

A log of wood is carried by the river to lower or

to higher ground. His body, carried by the river of time, enjoys or suffers the effects of past actions.

In past lives, while he still dwelt in ignorance, he created certain karmas. In this present life, he apparently enjoys or suffers their effects. But now he has reached illumination and no longer identifies himself with the body. His body moves among external objects, and he seems to enjoy or suffer the effects of past deeds—just like a man who is still ignorant. Really, however, he is established in Brahman, and merely inhabits the body as a calm, detached onlooker. His mind is clear of all distraction, and unmoved, like the pivot of a wheel.

He neither directs his senses toward external objects nor does he withdraw them. He stands like an onlooker, unconcerned. He does not desire the reward of his actions, for he is intoxicated by the Atman—that nectar of pure joy.

He who renounces the pursuit of any aim, either in this world or even in heaven itself, and remains absorbed in the Atman, is indeed the Lord Shiva Himself. He is the excellent knower of Brahman.

Even though he dwells in the body, he is eternally free. He has reached the blessed goal. He is the excellent knower of Brahman. When the body falls from him be comes merged in Brahman. He attains Brahman, the one without a second.

An actor remains the same person, even when dressed to play a part. The excellent knower of Brahman always remains Brahman, and nothing else.

When an illumined soul has attained oneness with Brahman, his body may wither and fall anywhere, like the shrivelled leaf of a tree. What does it matter? For he has already freed himself from body-consciousness, burning it away in the fire of knowledge.

The illumined soul lives eternally conscious of his oneness with Brahman. He tastes continually the joy of the Atman, the one without a second. In putting off this garment of skin, flesh and bone he does not have to consider if the place, the time or the circumstances are suitable.

◊ ◊ ◊

TO BE rid of the body is not liberation. Nor is a man set free by external forms of renunciation. Liberation is the cutting of the knot of ignorance in the heart.

Does a tree gain or lose anything because its leaf falls in a ditch and not in a river, or in sacred ground rather than in an open field?

The destruction of the body, the sense-organs, the life-breath and the brain is like the destruction of a leaf, a flower or a fruit. But the Atman, like the tree, still stands. The Atman is not affected—it is the real Self, the true Being, the embodiment of joy.

The scriptures define the Atman as "pure consciousness"—thereby showing that it is the eternal truth. Only the outer coverings die. They are made of ignorance, concealing the Atman.

"In truth," say the scriptures, "the Atman is immortal"—thereby showing that it stands inde-

structible among the things that change and
perish.

Stones, trees, grass, grain, straw, cloth and all
other substances, when burnt, are reduced to
ashes. The body, the senses, the vital forces, the
mind and all other physical manifestations, when
burnt by the fire of knowledge, become Brahman.

Darkness is merged in sunlight, its opposite. So
also, this apparent world is merged in Brahman.

When the jar is broken, the ether within it
becomes one with the surrounding ether. When
the coverings are destroyed, the knower of
Brahman becomes Brahman.

When milk is poured into milk, oil into oil,
water into water, they blend in absolute oneness.
So also the illumined seer, the knower of the
Atman, becomes one with the Atman.

∽　∽　∽

HE WHO has become liberated in this life gains
liberation in death and is eternally united with
Brahman, the Absolute Reality. Such a seer will
never be reborn.

He knows that he is one with Brahman, and
has burnt the coverings of ignorance in the fire of
this knowledge. Thus he has become Brahman.
How can Brahman be subject to birth?

Similarly, both bondage and liberation are the
fictions of our ignorance. They do not really exist
in the Atman. Just as a piece of rope remains
rope, whether or not we mistake it for a snake.
The imagined snake does not really exist in the
rope.

People speak of bondage and liberation—meaning the presence or absence of the covering veil of ignorance. But, in reality, Brahman has no covering. For there is none other than Brahman—the one without a second. If there were a covering, Brahman would not be unique. The scriptures admit no duality.

Bondage and liberation exist in the mind only, but the ignorant attribute them falsely to the Atman itself—just as they say the sun is darkened when it is merely covered by a cloud. But Brahman, the one without a second, the unchangeable reality, remains unattached. It is pure consciousness.

To imagine that the Atman can be bound or liberated is false. Both bondage and liberation are states of mind. Neither of them can be attributed to Brahman, the eternal reality.

Therefore both bondage and liberation are fictions of ignorance. They are not in the Atman. The Atman is infinite, without parts, beyond action. It is serene, stainless, pure. How can one imagine duality in Brahman, which is entire like the ether, without a second, the supreme reality?

There is neither birth nor death, neither bound nor aspiring soul, neither liberated soul nor seeker after liberation—this is the ultimate and absolute truth.

෴ ෴ ෴

TODAY I have revealed to you the supreme mystery. This is the inmost essence of all Vedanta, the crest-jewel of all the scriptures. I regard you as my own son—a true seeker after liberation. You are purged of all the taints of this dark age, and your mind is clear of desire.

ᔆ  ᔆ  ᔆ

HEARING these words of his master, the disciple prostrated himself before him with a reverent heart. Then, with his master's blessing, he went his way, set free from the bondage of ignorance.

The master also went his way, bringing purity to the whole world, his mind immersed in the ocean of absolute existence and joy.

ᔆ  ᔆ  ᔆ

IN THIS dialogue between master and disciple the true nature of the Atman has been set forth in a manner which seekers after liberation may easily understand.

May those spiritual aspirants who seek liberation, who have cleansed themselves of all the heart's impurities by the performance of selfless work, who are averse to worldly pleasures, who delight in the words of the scriptures, whose minds have entered peace—may they hospitably welcome this salutary teaching!

And to those who ignorantly wander the desert of this world, treading the circle of death and rebirth, weary, thirsty and oppressed by hot misery as if by the sun's fierce rays—may this teaching reveal Brahman, the one without a second, the giver of delight, the ocean of nectar which is spread before our very feet. May this teaching of Shankara bring success to their efforts and lead them to liberation.

Om . . . Peace—Peace—Peace.

# IV

# Shankara
# Raises and Answers
# Some Important Questions

*Prasna-Uttara-Malika*

"*A Garland of Questions and Answers*"


WHAT IS the best thing a spiritual aspirant can do?
    Carry out his guru's instructions.

What must be avoided?
    Deeds which lead us into greater ignorance of
    the truth.

Who is a guru?
    He who has found the truth of Brahman and is
    always concerned for the welfare of his dis-
    ciples.

What is the first and most important duty for a
    man of right understanding?
    To cut through the bonds of worldly desire.

How can one be liberated?
    By attaining the knowledge of Brahman.

Who, in this world, can be called pure?
  He whose mind is pure.

Who can be called wise?
  He who can discriminate between the real and
    the unreal.

What poisons the spiritual aspirant?
  Neglect of his guru's teachings.

For one who has achieved human birth, what is
    the most desirable objective?
  To realize that which is his ultimate good and
    to be constantly engaged in doing good to
    others.

What deludes a man like an intoxicating drink?
  Attachment to the objects of the senses.

What are thieves?
  The objects which steal our hearts away from
    the truth.

What causes the bondage of worldly desire?
  Thirst to enjoy these objects.

What is the obstacle to spiritual growth?
  Laziness.

What is the best weapon with which to subdue
    others?
  Sound reasoning.

Wherein lies strength?
  In patience.

Where is poison?
  Within the wicked.

What is fearlessness?
  Dispassion.

What is most to be feared?
To become possessed by your own wealth.

What is most rarely found among mankind?
Love for the Lord.

What are the evils most difficult to rid oneself of?
Jealousy and envy.

Who is dear to the Lord?
He who is fearless and takes away fear from others.

How does one attain liberation?
By practicing spiritual disciplines.

Who is most lovable?
The knower of Brahman.

How does one develop the power of discrimination?
Through service to an elder.

Who are elders?
Those who have realized the ultimate truth.

Who is truly wealthy?
He who worships the Lord with devotion.

Who profits from his life?
The humble man.

Who is a loser?
He who is proud.

What is the most difficult task for a man?
To keep his mind under constant control.

Who protects an aspirant?
His guru.

Who is the teacher of this world?
  The Lord.

How does one attain wisdom?
  By the grace of the Lord.

How is one liberated?
  Through devotion to the Lord.

Who is the Lord?
  He who leads us out of ignorance.

What is ignorance?
  The obstacle to the unfoldment of the Divine
    which is within us.

What is the ultimate Reality?
  Brahman.

What is unreal?
  That which disappears when knowledge
    awakes.

How long has ignorance existed?
  From a time without beginning.

What is unavoidable?
  The death of the body.

Whom should we worship?
  An incarnation of God.

What is liberation?
  The destruction of our ignorance.

Who is not to be trusted?
  He who lies habitually.

What is the strength of a holy man?
  His trust in God.

Who is a holy man?
  He who is forever blissful.

Who is free from sin?
  He who chants the name of the Lord.

What is the source of all the scriptures?
  The sacred syllable OM.

What carry us across the ocean of worldliness?
  The lotus feet of the Lord; they carry us like a
    great ship.

Who is bound?
  He who is attached to worldliness.

Who is free?
  He who is dispassionate.

How is heaven attained?
  The attainment of heaven is freedom from
    cravings.

What destroys craving?
  Realization of one's true self.

What is the gate to hell?
  Lust.

Who lives in happiness?
  He who has attained samadhi.

Who is awake?
  He who discriminates between right and wrong.

Who are our enemies?
  Our sense-organs, when they are uncontrolled.

Who are our friends?
  Our sense-organs, when they are controlled.

Who is poor?
  He who is greedy.

Who is totally blind?
  He who is lustful.

Who has overcome the world?
  He who has conquered his own mind.

What are the duties of a spiritual aspirant?
  To keep company with the holy, to renounce all
    thoughts of "me" and "mine", to devote
    himself to God.

Whose birth is blessed?
  His who does not have to be reborn.

Who is immortal?
  He who does not have to pass through another
    death.

When is one established in the ideal of renuncia-
    tion?
  When one knows that Atman and Brahman are
    one.

What is right action?
  Action which pleases the Lord.

In this world, what is the greatest terror?
  The fear of death.

Who is the greatest hero?
  He who is not terror-stricken by the arrows
    which shoot from the eyes of a beautiful girl.

Who is poor?
  He who is not contented.

What is meanness?
  To beg from someone who has less than you.

Whom should we honor?
  Him who does not beg from anyone.

Who, in this world, is truly alive?
  He whose character is free from blemish.

Who is awake?
  He who practices discrimination.

Who is asleep?
  He who lives in ignorance.

What roll quickly away, like drops of water from a
    lotus leaf?
  Youth, wealth and the years of a man's life.

Who are said to be as pure as the rays of the
    moon?
  Holy men.

What is hell?
  To live in slavery to others.

What is happiness?
  Detachment.

What is a man's duty?
  To do good to all beings.

What are worthless as soon as they are won?
  Honor and fame.

What brings happiness?
  The friendship of the holy.

What is death?
  Ignorance.

What is the most valuable thing?
  A gift given at the right time.

What disease lingers on until a man dies?
  A bad deed which has been hidden.

What should one strive for?
  To go on learning as long as one lives.

What should a man hate?
  Greed for the wives and the wealth of other
  men.

What should a man think of, day and night?
  He should think how transitory this world is.
  He should never think thoughts of lust.

What should we prize most dearly?
  Compassion, and friendship with the holy.

Whose heart do you fail to win even if you try
  your hardest?
  The heart of a fool or of a man who is afraid or
  stricken with grief or incapable of gratitude.

Who avoids the snares of the world?
  He who is truthful and who is able to remain
  unmoved by either pleasure or pain and all
  life's other pairs of opposites.

To whom do the gods themselves pay homage?
  To him who is compassionate.

Whom do all men respect?
  Him who is humble and speaks the truth so
  that it does good to others and makes them
  happy.

Who is blind?
  He who does evil deeds.

Who is deaf?
He who will not listen to good advice.

Who is dumb?
He who does not speak kind words when they are needed.

Who is a friend?
He who prevents another from doing evil.

What is man's best ornament?
His good character.

What is finished as quickly as lightning?
Friendship with bad men or women.

What qualities are rarest in this world?
To have the gift of speaking sweet words with compassion, to be learned without pride, to be heroic and also forgiving, to be rich without attachment to riches—these four are rare.

What is most to be deplored?
Miserliness in the wealthy.

What is to be praised?
Generosity.

Who is revered by the wise?
He who is humble.

Who wins glory for his entire family?
He who remains humble when endowed with greatness.

Who is the master of this world?
He whose words are sweet and beneficial and who follows the path of righteousness.

Who is never touched by any danger?
  He who follows the words of the wise and has
    his senses under control.

Where should one live?
  One should live with the holy.

What should a wise man refrain from uttering?
  Falsehoods and evil words against others.

What ought a man to remember?
  The sacred name of the Lord.

What are the enemies of the spiritual aspirant?
  Lust and greed.

What should a man protect from harm?
  A faithful wife and his power of discrimination.

What is the tree that fulfills all wishes?
  The teachings of the guru.